C000261479

Melanie Fennell is the author of *Overce...* *Overcoming Low Self-Esteem Handbook, Boo...* co-author (with Lee Brosan) of *An Introdu...* *Esteem*. She was a pioneer of cognitive behavioural therapy (CBT) in the UK, and is a Founding Fellow of the Oxford Cognitive Therapy Centre, an internationally recognised centre of excellence in CBT training, where she developed and led courses at Diploma and Masters level, as well as presenting many workshops and papers at major international conferences. As a member of research teams in the Oxford University Department of Psychiatry, Melanie has contributed to the development and evaluation of CBT and MBCT (Mindfulness-Based Cognitive Therapy) for a range of emotional problems, including depression, anxiety and PTSD. Her interest in low self-esteem grew out of this work. *Overcoming Low Self-Esteem* has become a classic of self-help literature, winning acclaim for the practical and user-friendly approach also to be found in the *Handbook*. It is recommended under the national Reading Well self-help scheme. In July 2002, Melanie was voted 'Most Influential Female UK Cognitive Therapist' by the membership of the British Association for Behavioural & Cognitive Therapies (BABCP), and in 2013 she was awarded an Honorary Fellowship by the Association.

The aim of the **Overcoming** series is to enable people with a range of common problems and disorders to take control of their own recovery programme.

Each title, with its specially tailored programme, is devised by a practising clinician using the latest techniques of cognitive behavioural therapy – techniques that have been shown to be highly effective in changing the way patients think about themselves and their problems.

Many books in the Overcoming series are recommended under the Reading Well scheme.

Titles in the series include:

THE OVERCOMING LOW SELF-ESTEEM HANDBOOK

A self-help guide using cognitive behavioural techniques

Melanie Fennell

ROBINSON

ROBINSON

First published in Great Britain in 2021 by Robinson

A CIP catalogue record for this book
is available from the British Library.

IMPORTANT NOTE
This book is not intended as a substitute for medical advice or treatment.
Any person with a condition requiring medical attention should consult a
qualified medical practitioner or suitable therapist.

ISBN: 978-1-47214-537-6

Typeset in Bembo by Initial Typesetting Services, Edinburgh
Printed and bound in Great Britain by Clays Ltd, Elcograf S.p.A.

Papers used by Robinson are from well-managed forests and
other responsible sources.

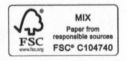

Robinson
An imprint of
Little, Brown Book Group
Carmelite House
50 Victoria Embankment
London EC4Y 0DZ

An Hachette UK Company
www.hachette.co.uk

www.littlebrown.co.uk

To my father, for his warmth, his resilience,
his humour, and his loving heart

Contents

Introduction:

How to Use this Handbook

This is a three-part self-help course for dealing with low self-esteem. It has two aims:

1. To help you develop a better understanding of the problem
2. To teach you the practical skills you will need in order to change

How the course works

The *Overcoming Low Self-Esteem Handbook* will help you understand how low self-esteem develops and what keeps it going, and then to make changes in your life so that you begin to feel more kindly and accepting towards yourself, more able to approach life with the confidence to be who you truly are.

This handbook is designed to help you work, either by yourself or with your healthcare practitioner, to overcome low self-esteem. With plenty of questionnaires, charts, worksheets and practical exercises, the three parts together make up a structured course.

Part One explains:

* What low self-esteem is
* How low self-esteem affects people

- How negative experiences affect people
- What keeps low self-esteem going

Part Two explains:

- How to recognise and deal with anxious predictions
- How to recognise and question self-critical thoughts
- How to identify your positive qualities
- How to gain a balanced view of yourself and start enjoying life
- How to treat yourself with respect, consideration and kindness

Part Three explains:

- What Rules for Living are
- How to change your Rules for Living
- How to recognise and change your central beliefs about yourself
- How to draft and fine-tune an Action Plan for the future

How long will the course take?

Each part of the handbook will probably take at least two or three weeks to work through – but do not worry if you feel that you need to give each one extra time. Some things can be understood and changed quite quickly, but others take longer. You will know when you are ready to move on. Completing the entire course could take only two to three months – or it could take longer. This will depend on how quickly you wish to work. Take your time and go at the pace that suits you best, allowing new learning to sink in, building on what you discover at each stage, and so gradually developing a new, more kindly, respectful and accepting view of yourself.

Getting the most from the course

Here are some tips to help you get the most from the handbook:

- It is not a priceless antique – it is a practical tool. So, feel free not only to write on the worksheets and charts, but also to underline and highlight things, and to write comments and questions in the margins. By the time you have finished with the handbook, it should look well and truly used.

- As well as worksheets, you will also find lots of space in the main text. This is for you to write down your thoughts and ideas, and your responses to the questions. Writing things down helps them to sink in. This makes them easier to remember in the long run and you can refer back to them at times when you are perhaps feeling stressed or unwell or tired, or your confidence has taken a knock.

- As well as copies in the book, you will also find all the worksheets and charts available for download from www.overcoming.co.uk.

- Each part of the handbook builds on what has already been covered. So, what you learn when working with one part will help you when you come to the next. It's quite possible simply to dip in and out, but you may get the most out of the course if you follow it through systematically, step by step, taking whatever time you need to feel the benefit of your work at each stage. Think of this as a gesture of respect and kindness towards yourself – you are worth it.

- Keep an open mind and be willing to explore new ideas and skills. Be alert to new possibilities (rather than letting old thinking habits automatically rule them out) and see if you can bring a sort of friendly curiosity to your investigations. It's important not just to think about things or talk about them, but to be ready to put new ideas into practice on a day-to-day basis and carefully note the results. Direct experience is the best teacher.

- The handbook will sometimes ask you to think about painful issues. This takes courage, but if low self-esteem is distressing you and restricting your life, it really is worth making the effort to overcome it. The rewards will be substantial.

- You will probably get the most out of the course if you are willing to set aside time each day to do the practical exercises – 20 to 30 minutes daily if you can.

- Try to answer all the questions and do the exercises, even if you have to come back to some of them later. There may be times when you get stuck and can't think how to take things forward. If this happens, don't get angry with yourself or give up. Just put the handbook aside and come back to it later, when you are feeling more relaxed

- You will almost certainly experience ups and downs as you work through the handbook, especially if your self-esteem has been low for some time. There is no need to be disheartened if you hit a rough patch – it's a normal part of trying to tackle any difficult problem. In fact, although rough patches and setbacks can be painful, if you carefully observe exactly what happened, you will learn a great deal about how your low self-esteem works and how to overcome it, step by step.

- You may find it helpful to work through the handbook with a friend or supporter. Two heads are often better than one. And you may be able to encourage each other to persist, even when one of you is finding it hard.

- At the end of each Section, before you move on to the next, take a moment to look over what you have done. While what you have learned is still fresh in your mind, use a Thoughts and Reflections Sheet to write down anything in that Section that has been particularly interesting or helpful to you – new ideas, new understandings, new ways of tackling your low self-esteem. You will find these sheets at the end of each

Section, and also at the back of the handbook. (You can also download them from www.overcoming.co.uk).
- Reread the handbook. You may get more out of it once you've had a chance to think about some of the ideas and put them into practice for a little while.

A NOTE OF CAUTION

This handbook will not help everyone who has low self-esteem. If you find that focusing on self-esteem is actually making you feel worse instead of better, or if your negative beliefs about yourself are so strong that you cannot even begin to use the ideas and practical skills described, you may be suffering from clinical depression. The recognised signs of clinical depression include:

- Constantly feeling sad, down, depressed or empty
- General lack of interest in what's going on around you
- A big increase or decrease in your appetite and weight
- A marked change in your sleep patterns
- Noticeable speeding up or slowing down in your movements and how you go about things
- Feeling of being tired and low in energy
- An intense sense of guilt or worthlessness
- Difficulty in concentrating and making decisions
- A desire to hurt yourself or a feeling that you might be better off dead

If you have had five or more of these symptoms (including low mood or loss of interest) for two weeks or more, you should seek professional help from a doctor, counsellor or psychotherapist. There is nothing shameful about seeking this sort of professional help – any more than there is

---

anything shameful about taking your car to a garage if it is not working as it should or going to see a lawyer if you have legal problems. It simply means taking your journey towards self-knowledge and self-acceptance with the help of a friendly guide, rather than striking out alone.

PART ONE:

Understanding Low Self-Esteem

SECTION 1:

What is Low Self-Esteem?

This section will help you to understand:

- what low self-esteem is
- whether you have low self-esteem
- how we develop beliefs about ourselves
- how low self-esteem affects a person
- how low self-esteem affects our lives
- how low self-esteem is linked to other problems
- how the impact of low self-esteem varies

What is low self-esteem?

Self-esteem refers to the overall beliefs or opinions we have about ourselves, and the value we place on ourselves as people. The tone of these may be negative or positive. When the tone is positive, this reflects broadly healthy self-esteem. Note that 'healthy self-esteem' does *not* mean a view of yourself as unrealistically positive as your current view of yourself may be unrealistically negative. You do not have to think you're wonderful, and everything you do is perfect. Rather, healthy self-esteem means having a *balanced* view of yourself, recognising that (like every other human being) you are a mix of strengths and weaknesses. Healthy self-esteem means being able to accept yourself just as you are, warts and all. At the heart of this is the sense that it's OK to be you. In contrast, people with

9

low self-esteem will have generally negative self-beliefs. They will tend to ignore or discount strengths, talents and good qualities and instead to focus on their flaws, their weaknesses, their mistakes, and the times they fall short. Self-critical thinking comes easily to them and bolsters their negative beliefs about themselves.

Look at the following statements and write 'N' next to the ones that sound negative.

a. 'I am comfortable with myself as I am.' _____

b. 'I'm useless.' _____

c. 'Nothing I do matters.' _____

d. 'I'm a good person.' _____

e. 'The things I do are worthwhile.' _____

f. 'I'm worthless.' _____

g. 'I am weak and inferior to other people.' _____

h. 'I appreciate and respect myself.' _____

i. 'I'm important to the people around me.' _____

j. 'I dislike myself.' _____

Do any of the negative statements sound familiar? Perhaps you have had some of these feelings yourself? To find out more, work through the next exercise.

Do I have low self-esteem?

Take a look at the ten statements below. Put a tick next to each question in the column that best reflects how you feel about yourself. Be honest – there are no right or wrong answers, simply tell the truth about how you see yourself.

	Yes, definitely	Yes, mostly	Yes, some-times	No, mostly	No, not at all
My experience in life has taught me to value and appreciate myself					
I have a good opinion of myself					
I treat myself well and look after myself properly					
I like myself					
I give as much weight to my qualities, skills, assets and strengths as I do to my weaknesses and flaws					
I feel good about myself					
I feel worthy of other people's attention and time					
It's OK for me to care for myself and to enjoy the good things in life					
My expectations of myself are no more rigid or exacting than my expectations of other people					
I am kind and encouraging towards myself, rather than being self-critical					

If your answers to these statements are not mainly 'Yes, definitely', then this book could be useful to you. If you're troubled by self-doubt, if your thoughts about yourself are often unkind and critical, or if you have difficulty in feeling that you have any true worth or that you deserve happiness, these are signs that your self-esteem is low. And low self-esteem may be having a painful and damaging effect on your life.

How does low self-esteem affect a person?

Negative beliefs about ourselves can be expressed in many ways (such as how we look and behave) and it's useful to learn how to recognise these outward signs.

If you think you have low self-esteem, you could consider yourself at this point. But you may find it easier to start by thinking about someone you know who you think has low self-esteem. This is because, when we try to look at ourselves, it is often difficult to get a clear view – we are too close to see the problem clearly.

Think about the person you have chosen. What are the signs and signals, the tell-tale clues that tell you this person has low self-esteem? Remember in as much vivid detail as you can a recent time when you met – see them in your mind's eye, hear them with your mind's ear. You may find it helpful to think of more than one person so a blank worksheet has been provided at the back of the book for you to use, and you will find more on the Overcoming website.

1. **What did you talk about?** (For example, did you hear lots of apologies, or a lot of self-criticism, self-blame or self-doubt?)

   _____

   _____

   _____

   _____

2. **How did the person behave?** (Did he or she sit hunched over, looking down? Did he or she speak in a hushed voice, or avoid making eye contact? Or did you perhaps have the feeling he or she was putting on a front – working hard to appear cheerful, for example, or trying too hard to please instead of relaxing and being natural?)

_____

_____

_____

_____

3. **What sort of mood was the person in?** (For example, did he or she seem sad, shy, anxious, ashamed, hopeless, frustrated or angry?)

_____

_____

_____

_____

4. **How was the person's body state?** (For example, did he or she seem tired, low in energy, restless or tense?)

_____

_____

_____

_____

This exercise shows how holding negative beliefs about yourself can affect thinking, behaviour, emotions and body sensations. Now that you have got an idea of what to look out for, ask yourself: If I was observing myself in the same way, what would I notice? What would be the tell-tale signs of low self-esteem in *my* case?

Thoughts:

_____

_____

_____

_____

_____

Behaviour:

_____

_____

_____

_____

_____

Emotions:

_____

_____

_____

_____

_____

Body state:

_____

_____

_____

_____

How does low self-esteem affect our lives?

Just as low self-esteem is reflected in many aspects of a person, so it has an impact on many areas of life.

Tick the statements below that most closely match how you feel.

Work (include study here if it's relevant to you)

☐ a. 'I work late nearly every night, but I still don't get half the things done I need to.'

☐ b. 'My parents are disappointed that I haven't done better.'

☐ c. 'I put in as much as I have to do for my work and no more. I sometimes think I could do something more demanding, but I'm a bit worried about having to learn new skills.'

☐ d. 'I thought about applying for a new job, but I know I probably won't get it, so I'm better off staying where I am.'

Personal relationships

☐ a. 'If someone criticises something I do, I always feel terrible.'

☐ b. 'I'm not very good in a group of people – I can't think what to say and often blush or stammer when I start to speak.'

☐ c. 'I sometimes find myself apologising for something that wasn't actually my fault.'

☐ d. 'I usually drink too much at social events to help me relax. If I didn't, I'd probably just stand in a corner feeling shy and awkward.'

Self-care

- ☐ a. 'I know I ought to take time off work when I'm sick, but I worry that I'll let my workmates down.'
- ☐ b. 'My hair's a mess and I could do with some new clothes.'
- ☐ c. 'I smoke a lot, and eat too many sweet things, especially when I'm stressed out or a bit down.'
- ☐ d. 'People tell me I obsess about the way I look but I'm worried about not being as attractive as possible all the time.'

Leisure activities

- ☐ a. 'I know I ought to do more exercise, but I don't dare join my local gym because everyone else there is really fit.'
- ☐ b. 'I'd like to join an art class, but I don't have any talent, so I'd just make a fool of myself.'
- ☐ c. 'I'd love to have a facial or a massage, but I'd feel guilty about spending money on myself.'
- ☐ d. 'I find it hard to sit down and relax – there's always something that needs doing in the house.'

Now let's look at your answers and see how low self-esteem may be affecting your life.

Work or study

If you ticked **a** or **b** you may be a real perfectionist and relentlessly work yourself hard. Nothing is good enough. You may not give yourself credit for your achievements or believe that good results come from your own skill and abilities.

If you ticked c or d you may have a pattern of avoiding challenges for fear of failing. People with low self-esteem often perform below their potential.

Personal relationships

If you ticked a you may be oversensitive to criticism and disapproval – inclined to feel it must be justified.

If you ticked b you may suffer from extreme self-consciousness, which may stop you expressing yourself. It could even make you want to back away from social situations altogether.

If you ticked c you may be so eager to please that you always put others first, no matter what the cost to yourself.

If you ticked d you may try to appear lively and confident but, underneath, you worry that if you don't behave in this way people will find you boring and won't want to know you.

Self-care

If you ticked a, b or c then you may not take proper care of yourself because you don't feel that you deserve to be looked after.

If you ticked d you may spend hours perfecting every detail of how you look, convinced that this is the only way to be attractive to other people.

Leisure activities

If you ticked a or b you may avoid any leisure activity in which there is a risk of being judged.

If you ticked c or d you may have an underlying belief that you do not deserve rewards, treats or any time to relax and enjoy yourself.

How is low self-esteem linked to other problems?

What looks like low self-esteem is sometimes purely **a reflection of current mood**. People whose mood is very low, whatever the reason for that, almost always see themselves in a painfully negative light. As their mood lifts, their sense of themselves may come back into balance without needing further work.

Alternatively, low self-esteem can be **a consequence of** other problems, such as:

- relationship difficulties
- financial hardship
- severe stress
- chronic pain or illness
- anxiety, constant debilitating worry, or panic attacks
- depression itself, when it is seen as a sign of personal weakness or inadequacy

All these problems can undermine confidence and lead to loss of self-esteem. In this case, tackling the root problem may provide the most effective solution. People who learn to manage anxiety or panic attacks, for example, often regain their confidence without needing to do much work on low self-esteem in its own right. If this is your situation, you may still find some useful ideas in this handbook to help you restore your belief in yourself. It could also be worth consulting other titles in the 'Overcoming' series to see whether any of them address your problems directly.

Finally, lasting low self-esteem can sometimes be **a factor contributing to the development of other problems**, such as:

- depression
- suicidal thoughts
- eating disorders (e.g. anorexia or binge-eating)
- substance abuse
- extreme shyness

If this is the case for you, if the difficulties you are currently experiencing seem to spring from an underlying sense of low self-esteem, then working with those difficulties may well be useful, but is unlikely to produce real change in your view of yourself. To make lasting changes, you probably need to tackle the issue of low self-esteem in its own right. In this case, you could benefit greatly from using this handbook as a guide to working systematically on your beliefs about yourself, undermining the old negative views and building up new, more helpful perspectives.

How does the impact of low self-esteem vary?

You may be a person who is generally self-confident but suffers from occasional moments of self-doubt in particularly challenging situations. Or you may be someone who is constantly tormented by self-criticism and finds it hard to think of anything good about yourself. Or of course you may be somewhere in between these two extremes.

Imagine how you would feel in the following situations and put a cross on the line, between 0 (calm and confident) and 10 (extremely anxious):

1. You are about to be interviewed for a new job.

0   5   10

2. You are asking someone out for a first date.

0   5   10

3. You have been invited to a big party where you will know only a few people.

0   5   10

19

4. You have been sold a defective product and you need to get a refund from the supplier.

0   5   10

5. Someone who works for your firm has been coming in late every day and you have to reprimand him or her.

0   5   10

If most of your crosses are towards the extreme left, your self-doubt is probably only triggered in certain situations and you can generally manage it without serious distress or difficulty. When you have difficulties in life, you usually see them as problems to be solved, rather than as a sign that there is something fundamentally wrong with you as a person. You have some kinder and more accepting alternative perspectives on yourself, which balance out self-doubt triggered by challenging situations. If this describes you, it should be possible for you quite easily to identify the situations that are problematic, and to learn rapidly how to deal constructively with your doubts. Thus, this handbook will be useful mainly in helping to fine-tune an already strong sense of self-confidence.

If on the other hand most of your crosses are towards the extreme right, you may suffer from highly distressing self-doubt and self-criticism almost all the time. Your fears and negative beliefs about yourself may cause you to miss opportunities, avoid challenges, and follow self-defeating and self-destructive patterns of behaviour. You tend to see difficulties in life as being central to your true self ('This is me.' 'This is who I am.'). So, it is hard to step back far enough to see things clearly, or to work systematically to change things for the better. Working through this handbook on your own may not enable you to dislodge your negative self-beliefs. You may also need help from a professional therapist. If you like the approach described in this book, then perhaps a cognitive-behavioural therapist might be helpful to you.

Most people fall somewhere between these two extremes. If you are in this middle range, this handbook will be particularly useful. You will be aware of your low self-esteem and wish to do something about it. You will also be able to stand back from the way you habitually see yourself and search for alternative perspectives. As you work through the book, you will begin to understand how your negative opinions developed, use close self-observation to change old thinking patterns, and replace those unhelpful beliefs with a new, more kindly, respectful and accepting view of yourself. You may be able to do this on your own, or you might find it helpful to work with a supporter (for example, a good friend), or a therapist.

SUMMARY

1. Self-esteem reflects how you think about yourself, the judgements you make about yourself, and the value you place on yourself as a person.
2. 'Low self-esteem' means having a poor opinion of yourself, judging yourself harshly and feeling you have little worth or value.
3. In contrast, healthy self-esteem means having a balanced view of yourself which both accepts your human weaknesses and appreciates your strengths and good qualities.
4. At the heart of low self-esteem lie negative beliefs about yourself. These are reflected in your everyday thoughts, feelings and actions, and can affect many areas of life.

5. Low self-esteem can be an aspect, a cause or an effect of a whole range of other difficulties.

6. The extent to which low self-esteem disrupts daily life varies from person to person.

SECTION 2:

Understanding How Low Self-Esteem Develops

This section will help you understand:

- where beliefs about ourselves come from
- how low self-esteem develops
- how negative experiences affect people
- how negative experiences lead to your Bottom Line
- what biased thinking is
- what your Rules for Living are

Where do beliefs about ourselves come from?

At the heart of self-esteem lie your central beliefs about yourself. You may think of these beliefs as facts, reflections of the real truth about you. But beliefs are actually opinions rather than facts – and it's important to remember that opinions can be mistaken, biased, inaccurate or just plain wrong. And opinions can be changed.

Most people's ideas about themselves are based on the experiences they've had in their lives and the messages they've received about the kind of people they are.

If your experiences have generally been positive and affirming – if good things have happened to you, if you've been surrounded by loving family and friends, if you've done well at school and at work, been praised for your successes and your talents – then your beliefs about yourself are likely to be positive and affirming too.

If your experiences have been mixed – if for example you weren't the most popular person at school but then blossomed in your first job, if your first real love let you down but you then met a supportive and loving partner – then you may have a good opinion of yourself in some circumstances, but feel bad about yourself in others.

However, if your experiences have been generally negative and undermining – at home as you were growing up, at school, at work, in relationships – then you may well have negative and undermining beliefs about yourself; in other words, low self-esteem.

As you read through this section of the handbook, think about how the ideas might apply to you personally:

- What do you recognise from your own life?
- What helps you to make sense of how you feel about yourself?
- Which of the stories ring bells for you?
- What are the experiences that have contributed to low self-esteem in your own particular case?

On paper or an electronic equivalent (you could use a 'Thoughts and Reflections' sheet for this), note down anything that occurs to you as you read – ideas, memories, hunches. The aim is to help you to understand why it is that you have low self-esteem. You will discover that your ideas about yourself are an understandable reaction to what has happened to you – that is, anyone with your life experience would probably hold similar views.

You will begin to see how conclusions you reached about yourself (perhaps many years ago) have influenced the way you have thought and felt and acted over time. This understanding is the first vital step towards change. Once you understand how your low self-esteem works, you can begin to observe it do what it does in real time, as it actually happens. You will begin to see how these compelling and painful ideas are in fact nothing more than unhelpful old habits of thought. You will learn to say to yourself 'Oh look, there it is again', rather than accepting without question that the voice of low self-esteem tells the truth. And once you can say 'Oh look, there it is again', you have already stepped back a little from this unkind, self-defeating thinking, and begun to discover that you no longer need to engage with it, get sucked into it, or believe what it says. As one person said: 'Not "I am a failure" anymore, but "Here I go, *thinking* I am a failure".' You have begun your journey towards creating a new sense of self-acceptance, a new perspective on yourself.

How does low self-esteem develop?

These are the ingredients that lead to low self-esteem:

LOW SELF-ESTEEM: A Map of the Territory

(Early) Experience
Events, relationships, living conditions which have implications for your ideas about yourself e.g. rejection; neglect; abuse; criticism and punishment; lack of praise, interest, warmth; being the 'odd one out'

↓

The Bottom Line
Assessment of your worth/value as a person
Conclusions about yourself, based on experience: *'This is the kind of person I am'*
e.g. *I am bad; I am worthless; I am stupid; I am not good enough*

↓

Rules For Living
Guidelines, policies or strategies for getting by, given that you assume the Bottom Line to be true
Standards against which self-worth can be measured e.g. *I must always put others first; If I say what I think, I will be rejected; Unless I do everything to the highest possible standard, I will achieve nothing*

↓

Trigger Situations
Situations in which your Rules for Living are (or may be) broken
e.g. being rejected, the possibility of failing, feeling that you might lose control

This flowchart shows how **Negative Early Experiences** can lead to a negative **Bottom Line** (negative beliefs about yourself). Because the **Bottom Line** seems to be true, rather than just a belief or an opinion, we then adopt **Rules for Living** which are designed to help us get by, but in fact keep us stuck in low self-esteem. Then, when we find ourselves in a relevant **Trigger Situation** (for example, when we believe we have failed or think we might lose control), the **Bottom Line** is activated and we feel as if our negative beliefs about ourselves are indeed true ('There you are, I *knew* it').

How do negative experiences affect people?

Beliefs about ourselves (and indeed about other people and about life) are all learned. They have their roots in experience. Your beliefs about yourself are conclusions you have reached on the basis of what has happened to you. This means that, however unhelpful or outdated they may now be, they are nonetheless understandable – there was a time when they made perfect sense, given what was going on in your life.

You can learn in many ways – from direct experience, from your own observation, from the media and social media, from listening to what people around you say and watching what they do. Important experiences, which may help to form your beliefs about yourself, often (though not necessarily) occur early in life. What you saw, heard and experienced in childhood and as you were growing up – in your family, at school and among your friends – will have influenced your thinking in ways that may have persisted to the present day.

COMMON NEGATIVE EXPERIENCES

As a child:

1. Were you regularly punished, neglected or abused?
2. Did you fail to meet your parents' expectations, or were you compared unfavourably to others?
3. Were you teased, excluded or bullied by other children, face to face or online?
4. Were you on the receiving end of other people's stress or distress?
5. Was your family or social group struggling with adversity (e.g. financial hardship or illness), or was it a target for hostility or prejudice?
6. Did you lack enough of the things you needed in order to develop a secure, healthy sense of self-esteem (e.g. praise, affection, warmth or interest)?
7. Were you the 'odd one out' at home?
8. Were you the 'odd one out' at school?

Later on, as an adult:

9. Did you experience bullying at work, an abusive relationship, long-term stress or hardship, major changes or disruptions in your life, or serious traumatic events?
10. Did you lose things that were important to your sense of self-worth, for example losing youth, health, good looks or earning capacity?

Let's look at each of these issues in more detail, with the stories of some real people who have experienced these problems in their own lives. As you read, remember to ask yourself how does this relate to *my* life experience?

1 Regular punishment, neglect or abuse

If children are treated badly, they often assume that they must have somehow deserved it. If you were frequently punished (especially if the punishment was excessive, unpredictable or made no sense to you), if you were neglected, abandoned or abused, these experiences will have influenced the way you see yourself.

BRIONY'S STORY

Briony was adopted by her father's brother and his wife after both her parents were killed in a car crash when she was seven. Her new step-parents already had two older daughters. Briony became the family scapegoat. Everything that went wrong was blamed on her. Briony was a loving little girl, who liked to please people. She tried desperately to be good, but nothing worked. Every day she faced new punishments. She was deprived of contact with friends, made to give up music — which she loved — and was forced to do more than her fair share of work around the house. Briony became more and more confused. She could not understand why everything she did was wrong.

One night, when she was eleven, Briony's stepfather came silently into her room in the middle of the night. He put his hand over her mouth and raped her. He told her that she was dirty and disgusting, that she had asked for it, and that if she told anyone what had happened, no one would believe her, because they all knew she was a filthy little liar. Afterwards, she crept around the house in terror. No one seemed to notice or care. Briony's doubts about herself crystallised into a firm belief at that point. She was bad. Other people could see it and would treat her accordingly.

2 Failing to meet parental expectations, being unfavourably compared to others

If you were treated as if nothing you did was good enough, people focused on your mistakes at the expense of your successes, teased you, or made you feel small, all these experiences may have left you with the sense that there was something fundamentally wrong with you.

RAJIV'S STORY

Rajiv's father worked in a bank. He had never realised his ambitions to rise to a manager's position and put this down to the fact that his parents had failed to support him during his years at school. They had never seemed particularly interested in what he was doing, and it was easy to skip school and neglect his homework. He was determined not to make the same mistake with his own children. Every day, at the supper table, he would question them about what they had learned. Everyone had to have an answer, and the answer had to be good enough. They were repeatedly reminded of a cousin's hard work and his success in life.

Rajiv remembered dreading the sight of his father's car in the drive when he came home. It meant another grilling. He was sure his mind would go blank and he would be unable to think of anything to say. When this happened, his father's face would fall in disappointment. Rajiv could see that he was letting his father down. He felt he fully deserved the close questioning that followed. 'If you can't do better than this,' his father would say, 'you'll never get anywhere in life.' In his heart of hearts, Rajiv agreed. It was clear to him that he was not good enough: he would never make it.

3 Being teased, excluded or bullied by other children, face to face or online

Children and young people can be powerfully influenced, not only by their parents' standards, but also by the expectations of others of the same age. Particularly during adolescence, when you are developing your own personality and sexual identity, the pressure to fit in can be very strong. It may be reinforced by idealised images of celebrity in the press and social media. This is how you should look, what you should buy, what you should want out of life. Feeling that you are failing to make the grade can be very painful and lonely and may lead to low self-esteem.

EVIE'S STORY

Evie was an attractive, sturdy, energetic girl who enjoyed sport and loved dancing. She grew up at a time when the ideal body shape for women was to be tall and extremely slender. Although she was not at all overweight, Evie's natural body shape was not even close to this fashionable ideal. Her mother tried to boost her confidence by telling her that she was 'well built'. This clumsy attempt to help her to feel OK about herself backfired. 'Well built' was not what she was supposed to be. Evie was ignored by the popular girls at school. She knew about other girls who had been cyberbullied for their looks, and hardly dared to look at social media. Even her friends bought into the airbrushed celebrity look. They were passionate about fashion and spent hours shopping, trying on clothes, experimenting with make-up, and practising the required posture and expression for selfies. Evie would join them but felt horribly awkward and self-conscious. Every photo and mirror showed how far her body failed to meet the ideal. Her broad shoulders and rounded hips were just completely wrong.

Evie decided to diet. In the first two weeks, she lost a couple of kilos. Her friends thought she looked great. Evie was delighted. She continued to restrict her eating and to lose weight. But somehow, no matter how hard she tried, she could never be thin enough. And she was constantly hungry. In the end, she gave in and began to eat normally again, and then to overeat. This was the beginning of a lifelong pattern of alternately dieting and overeating. Evie was never happy with her physical self. As far as she was concerned, she was fat and ugly.

4 Being on the receiving end of other people's stress or distress

Even in loving families, changes in circumstances can sometimes create distress that has a lasting impact on children. Parents who are stressed, unhappy or distracted may have little patience with normal naughtiness, or with a young child's natural lack of self-control and skill.

JACK'S STORY

Jack was an energetic, adventurous, curious little boy. He had very little fear and, even as a toddler, was climbing trees and plunging into deep water without a second thought. His mother used to say she needed eyes in the back of her head to keep track of him. Jack's parents were proud of his adventurousness and found him funny and endearing.

When he was three, however, twin babies arrived. At the same time, Jack's father lost his job and had to take work at a much lower rate of pay. The family moved from a house with a garden to a small apartment on the fourth floor of a large block. With two new babies, things were chaotic. Jack's father felt his job loss keenly, and became gloomy and irritable. His mother was constantly tired. In the confined space of the apartment, there was nowhere for Jack's energy to go, and his interest and curiosity only made a mess.

He became a target for anger and frustration. Because he was only little, he did not understand why this change had happened. He tried hard to sit quietly and keep out of trouble, but again and again he ended up being shouted at and sometimes smacked. It was no longer possible to be himself without being told he was a naughty, disobedient boy. Even as an adult, whenever he met with disapproval or criticism, he still felt the old sense of despair. No one would ever want him — he was just all wrong.

5 *Belonging to a family or social group struggling with adversity, or a target for hostility or prejudice*

Your beliefs about yourself may not simply be based on how you personally were treated. Sometimes low self-esteem is partly caused by the way a person and his or her family live, or by his or her identity as a member of a group. If, for example, your family was very poor, if your parents had serious difficulties which meant the neighbours looked down on them, if you were a member of a racial, cultural or religious group which was a focus for hostility, these experiences may have left you feeling inferior to other people.

AARON'S STORY

Aaron was the middle one of seven children, in a family of travellers. He was brought up by his mother and his maternal grandmother and had no long-term father figure. Aaron's grandmother, a striking woman with bleached hair, coped by drinking. Aaron had clear memories of being rushed through the streets to school, his grandmother pushing two babies crammed into a buggy, the older children and another whining toddler trailing behind. Lack of money meant that all the children wore second-hand clothes, which were passed down from one to the next. Their sweatshirts were grubby, their shoes scuffed, their faces smudged, their hair standing on end. Every so often, the grandmother would stop and screech at the older children to hurry up.

What stuck in Aaron's mind was the faces of people coming in the opposite direction as they saw the family approaching. He would see their mouths twist, their disapproving frowns, their eyes looking away. He could hear their muttered comments to one another. The same happened when they reached the school. In the playground, other children and their parents kept away from him and his family.

Aaron's grandmother, too, was well aware of other people's attitudes. She was fiercely protective of the family, in her own way. She would shout and swear, calling names and screaming threats.

Throughout his schooldays, Aaron felt a deep sense of shame. He saw himself as a worthless outcast, whose best form of defence was attack. He was constantly fighting other kids, didn't concentrate in lessons, left with no qualifications, and spent his time with other young men operating on the fringes of the law. The only time he felt good about himself was when he had successfully broken the rules – perhaps stolen something without being caught or beaten someone up without reprisals.

6 Lacking what you needed in order to develop secure, healthy self-esteem (e.g. praise, affection, warmth, interest)

It is easy to see how abuse or prejudice could contribute towards someone feeling bad, inferior, weak or unlovable. But sometimes the important experiences are less obvious. If you had a fairly settled, normal childhood, how come you have so much trouble believing in your own worth?

Perhaps the problem was an *absence* of the day-to-day good things that make a person feel accepted and valued? Perhaps, for example, you did not receive *enough* interest, *enough* praise and encouragement, *enough* warmth and affection? Perhaps in your family, although there was no actual unkindness, love and appreciation were not directly expressed? If so, this could have influenced your ideas about yourself.

KATE'S STORY

Kate was brought up by elderly, middle-class parents. At heart, both were good people who tried their best to give their only daughter a sound start in life. However, they both had difficulty in openly expressing affection. Their only means of showing how much they loved her was by caring for her practical needs. So, they were good at ensuring that Kate did her homework, in seeing that she ate a balanced diet, that she was well dressed and had a good range of books and toys.

As she grew older, they made sure she went to a good school, took her to Girl Guides and swimming lessons, and paid for her to go on holiday with friends. But they almost never touched her – there were no cuddles, no kisses, no pet names. At first, Kate was hardly aware of this. But once she began to see how openly loving other families were, she began to experience a sad emptiness at home. She did her best to change things. She would take her father's hand as they walked along – but noticed how he would drop it as soon as he decently could. She would put her arms round her mother – and feel how she stiffened. She tried to talk about how she felt, but her parents quickly changed the subject.

Kate concluded that their behaviour must reflect something about her. Her parents did their duty by her, but no more. It must mean she was fundamentally unlovable.

7 Being the 'odd one out' at home

Another less obvious experience that can contribute to low self-esteem is the experience of being the 'odd one out'. Perhaps you were an artistic child in an academic family? Or you may have been an energetic, sporty child in a quiet family? Or perhaps you realised as you grew up that your sexual orientation or sense of your true gender might not be accepted or approved of by your more conventional parents and siblings? In each case, there was nothing particularly wrong with you, or with them, but for some reason you did not fit the family norm. Other family members may only have teased you in a good-natured way or perhaps expressed mild puzzlement. But you could still have ended up with a sense that being different from the norm means being odd, unacceptable or inferior.

LIN'S STORY

Lin was an exceptional artist. However, both her parents were teachers who believed that academic achievement was the most important thing in life. They were plainly delighted with her two older brothers, who did very well at school and became a doctor and a lawyer. Lin, however, was an average student. There was nothing particularly wrong with her schoolwork – she simply did not shine as her parents hoped she would. Her real talent lay in her hands and eyes. She could draw and paint, and her collages were full of energy and colour. Lin's parents tried to appreciate her artistic gifts, but they saw art and craft work as hobbies, essentially a waste of time. They never openly criticised her. But she could see how their faces lit up when they heard about her brothers' achievements, while showing little enthusiasm when she brought her artwork home. They always seemed to have more important things to do than look carefully at what she had done ('Very nice, dear').

Lin concluded that she was inferior to other, cleverer people. As an adult, she found it difficult to take pleasure in her artistic talent, tended to apologise for her work, and fell silent in the company of anyone she saw as more intelligent or educated than herself.

8 Being the 'odd one out' at school

In the same way that not fitting into your family can make it difficult to feel good about yourself, so being in some way different from others at school can lead people to see themselves as weird, alien or inferior. As we saw in Evie's case, school can be a demanding environment. We have to fit in and get along with all sorts of people, whether we like them or not. We may feel pressure to wear the right clothes, have the right haircut or mobile phone, listen to the right bands, get lots of 'likes' on social media. Children and young people who stand out from the group can be cruelly teased and excluded. For many children – whether it's having a different skin colour, wearing spectacles, being shy, having a different accent, being very good at schoolwork or being very slow to learn – being different means there must be something wrong with *them*. Did you feel like the 'odd one out' at school because of your appearance, personality or abilities?

CHRIS'S STORY

Chris's early childhood was happy. But he began to experience difficulties as soon as he went to school, because of undiagnosed dyslexia. While all the other children in the class seemed to be racing ahead with their reading and writing, he lagged behind. He just could not get the hang of it. He was assigned a teacher to give him special help and had to keep a special home reading record which was different from everyone else's.

Other children started to laugh at him and call him 'thicko' and 'dumbo'. He made up for this by becoming the class clown. He was the one who would always get involved in silly pranks. The teachers began to lose patience with him, and to label his difficulties laziness and attention-seeking. When his parents were called to the school yet again to discuss his behaviour, his comment to them was: 'What can you expect? I'm just stupid.'

9 Problems in adulthood

Although low self-esteem is often rooted in childhood or adolescent experiences, later experiences can also have a big impact. Even confident people, with strong positive views of themselves, can have their self-esteem weakened by things that happen later in life. Examples include being bullied at work, being trapped in an abusive marriage, being ground down by a long period of stress or financial hardship or experiencing a major trauma. Other less dramatic changes can also impact on self-esteem, if they involve the loss of things that have been central to feeling good about yourself (e.g. deteriorating health, fitness, looks or capacity to earn).

MIKE'S STORY

Mike was a fireman. As part of his job, he had attended many accidents and fires, and saved several people's lives. He had a stable, happy childhood and felt loved by both his parents. He saw himself as strong, and able to deal with anything life might throw at him. This was why he was able to remain outgoing and cheerful, despite his risky and demanding job.

One day, as he was driving down a busy street, a woman stepped off the pavement immediately in front of him and was caught under the wheels of his car. By the time he was able to stop, she had been fatally injured. Mike always carried a first aid kit, and he got out of the car to see what he could do. After a while, however, during which other people had called an ambulance and gathered round to help, he felt increasingly sick and shocked and retreated to his car.

Like many people who have suffered or witnessed horrific accidents, Mike later began to suffer symptoms of post-traumatic stress. He kept replaying the accident in his mind. He was tormented by guilt – he should have been able to stop the car; he should have stayed with the victim to the bitter end. He was constantly tense, irritable and miserable. Mike's usual way of coping with difficulties was to tell himself that life goes on, that he must put it behind him. Up until now, this had worked well for him. So, he tried not to think about what had happened. Unfortunately, this made it impossible for him to come to terms with it. He began to feel that his personality had changed. The fact that he had not been able to prevent the accident, that he had withdrawn to the car, and that he could not control his feelings meant that, far from being the strong, competent person he had believed himself to be, he was actually weak and inadequate – in fact, pathetic.

MARY'S STORY

Experiences in life do not have to be as dramatic as Mike's. More gradual losses and changes can have a substantial impact, if what is lost or changed is something on which a person has based his or her sense of worth. Mary, for example, was a thoughtful, sensitive person, very attuned to the needs of others and glad to help. She was always the one who took care of everybody else. She was praised as a child for this and came to see it as the essence of who she was. In fact, she loved doing it, and her caring nature and kind deeds were deeply appreciated by everyone who knew her. But as she grew older, her health, her strength and her energy gradually declined. She became less and less able to care for others in the practical ways she had done in the past. Rather than realising that, because of her kind heart, she still had much to offer in terms of attentive listening and loving support, Mary felt more and more downhearted. What use was she now? None whatsoever.

Connecting the past and the present: your Bottom Line

As people grow up, they continue to hear, in their minds, the voices of people who were important to them. Parents, grandparents, older brothers or sisters, teachers, child-minders, friends and schoolmates can all have a major impact on self-confidence and self-esteem. We may criticise ourselves in their exact, sharp tones, call ourselves the same unkind names.

We may experience emotions and body sensations from an earlier time in our lives and see images in our mind's eye of events that occurred many years ago. Lin, for example, when she submitted a painting for exhibition, would hear her mother's patient voice ('Well, I suppose if *you* like it, dear') and experience the same sinking feeling in her stomach that she experienced as a child. Jack, when in the best of spirits and full of energy, would suddenly catch a flash in his mind's eye of his father's shouting, angry face and feel instantly in the wrong.

Why is this? How come these events, which happened so long ago, still live on in our memories so vividly, and continue to influence how we feel and think and act in the present?

The answer lies in the way that our experiences have led us to make judgements about ourselves as people. These judgements form your self-esteem – what we will call the 'Bottom Line'. The Bottom Line is the view of yourself that lies at the heart of low self-esteem. It can often be summed up in a single sentence, beginning with the words, 'I am . . . '

To get a sense of what this means, look back over the stories you have just read and see if you can match the Bottom Lines on the left below with the names of the people on the right. Draw a line linking the name of each person with his or her Bottom Line (cover up the real answers just below before you do this):

I am stupid	Evie
I am bad	Mike
I am useless	Chris
I am fat and ugly	Briony
I am worthless	Kate
I am not good enough	Mary
I am unlovable	Lin
I am not important	Jack
I am pathetic	Aaron
I am all wrong	Rajiv

Here are their actual Bottom Lines:

Briony:	I am bad
Rajiv:	I am not good enough
Evie:	I am fat and ugly
Jack:	I am all wrong
Aaron:	I am worthless

Kate:	I am unlovable
Lin:	I am not important
Chris:	I am stupid
Mike:	I am pathetic
Mary:	I am useless

The negative ideas that these people developed about themselves made perfect sense to them, given their experiences. But, when you read their stories, did you agree with their opinions? Did *you* think that:

- Briony was bad?
- Rajiv was a failure?
- Evie was fat and ugly?
- Jack was all wrong?
- Aaron deserved to be an outcast?
- Kate was unlovable?
- Lin was unimportant?
- Chris was stupid?
- Mike was inadequate and weak – in a word, pathetic?
- Mary was useless?

As an outsider, you could probably see that Briony was not responsible for what her stepfather did to her, that Rajiv's father's own needs were clouding his judgement, that Evie's only shortcoming was not meeting a false ideal, that Jack's parents changed towards him because their difficult circumstances made them lose sight of his lovable qualities. You probably also realised that the disapproval Aaron attracted as a small child was not his fault, that it was Kate's parents' own limitations that prevented them from being more loving towards her, that Lin's parents' narrow standards prevented them from enjoying her artistic gifts, that Chris's slowness to learn was nothing to do with stupidity, that Mike's distress was an understandable reaction to a horrific event and not a sign of weakness or inadequacy, and that Mary was still the same caring person she had always been, even if her health now stopped her from expressing it in the same way.

Now think about your own view of yourself and the experiences that have fed into it while you were growing up and perhaps also later in your life. Use these questions to help you to put your own Bottom Line into words.

1. What do you say about yourself when you are being self-critical?

_____

_____

_____

_____

2. What names do you call yourself when you are angry and frustrated?

_____

_____

_____

_____

3. What were the words people in your life used to describe you when they were angry, or disappointed in you?

_____

_____

_____

_____

4. What messages about yourself did you pick up from your parents, other members of your family or your schoolmates and friends?

_____

_____

_____

_____

5. If you could express your Bottom Line in a single 'I am . . .' sentence, what would it be? Don't rush this – take a moment to see what comes to mind. You may find one Bottom Line, or you may discover more than one.

_____

_____

_____

_____

6. What experiences is this opinion based on? What comes to mind when you think back to when you first felt this way about yourself? Did a single event, or a series of events over time, form your ideas? Or was there a general atmosphere – perhaps of coldness or disapproval?

_____

_____

_____

_____

_____

Make a note of your ideas. You will be able to use this information later on to help you find a broader, more balanced and more compassionate perspective on yourself.

Understanding the origins of your low self-esteem is the first step towards change. You can probably see that the conclusions Briony and the others reached about themselves were based on misunderstandings about the meanings of their experiences – misunderstandings that made perfect sense at the time, given that they were children, with no adult knowledge on which to base a broader, more realistic view. Or, in Mike's case, too distressed to think straight about himself.

IT'S WORTH REMEMBERING

However powerful and convincing your Bottom Line may seem, it is usually biased and inaccurate, often because it is based on a child's eye view.

Think about your own Bottom Line.

- Are your own negative ideas about yourself based on similar misunderstandings?

_____

_____

_____

_____

_____

- Have you blamed yourself for something that was not your fault?

_____

_____

_____

_____

_____

- Have you taken responsibility for someone else's behaviour?

_____

_____

_____

_____

_____

- Have you seen specific problems (for example, difficulty asserting yourself) as a sign that you are a person of little worth?

_____

_____

_____

_____

_____

- Did you accept other people's standards and expectations before you were experienced enough to see their limitations and question them?

_____

_____

_____

_____

_____

- If another person had had your experiences, would you judge them as negatively as you do yourself? Or would you come to different conclusions?

_____

_____

_____

_____

_____

- How would you understand and explain what happened to you, if it had happened to someone you respected and cared about rather than to yourself?

_____

_____

_____

_____

_____

You may not find it easy at first to answer these questions, so take your time and come back to them as many times as you find helpful.

Once the Bottom Line is in place, it can be very difficult to realise that in fact it is just an idea that you picked up a long time ago, an old thinking habit – something you can learn to stand back from, question and test. This is because the Bottom Line is strengthened by biased thinking, which makes you home in on anything that supports your negative conclusions, while encouraging you to screen out anything that does not support them.

What is biased thinking?

Biased thinking means always looking at yourself and interpreting what you see in a negative way.

Biased perception (focusing on weaknesses and ignoring strengths)

If your self-esteem is low, you are probably quick to notice anything about yourself that you do not like. It could be a physical feature (e.g. 'My eyes are too small'), your character (e.g. 'I wish I wasn't so shy') or a mistake that you make (e.g. 'Not again. How *could* I be so stupid?'). On the other hand, you may automatically screen out anything good about yourself, anything that is not consistent with your negative belief. So, whenever you think about your looks, character or behaviour, you home in on your weaknesses and ignore your strengths. The end result is that you keep focusing on what you think is wrong with you, and not on what is right.

To see how this applies to you, think back over the last week or two and write down three occasions when you homed in on a weakness or ignored a strength (there is an extra page at the back of this book if you need it):

1. _____

_____

_____

_____

_____

_____

2. _____

_____

_____

_____

_____

_____

3. _____

_____

_____

_____

_____

Biased interpretation (always seeing the downside)

Low self-esteem not only unbalances what you notice about yourself, it also changes the way you interpret what happens to you. If something does not go well, you may use it as the basis for a general judgement about yourself (e.g. 'Typical, I always get it wrong'). So even quite small mistakes can appear to reflect your entire worth as a person. Even neutral and positive experiences can be twisted to fit a biased, negative view of yourself. For example, if someone compliments you on looking well, you may think 'Hmm, then I must have been looking pretty bad up till now'. Or you may dismiss the compliment altogether (e.g. 'They were only being kind – they just feel sorry for me'). This sort of biased interpretation always favours self-criticism, rather than encouragement, self-acceptance or self-appreciation.

Write down three recent occasions when you twisted something that happened to fit your view of yourself (again, there is an extra page at the back of the handbook if you need it):

1. _____

_____

_____

_____

2. _____

_____

_____

_____

3. _____

_____

_____

_____

IT'S WORTH REMEMBERING...

Biased perception and biased interpretation work together to support and strengthen your Bottom Line.

The end result

Negative beliefs and biased thinking trap you in a vicious circle, as you can see illustrated below. Given your negative beliefs about yourself, you tend to predict that things will turn out badly. This assumption makes you sensitive to any sign that things are indeed turning out badly. In addition, no matter how things *do* turn out, you are likely to see them in a negative light. Because of this, your memories of what happened will also be negatively biased. This strengthens your negative beliefs about yourself and makes you even more likely to predict the worst in future.

Biased thinking: a vicious circle

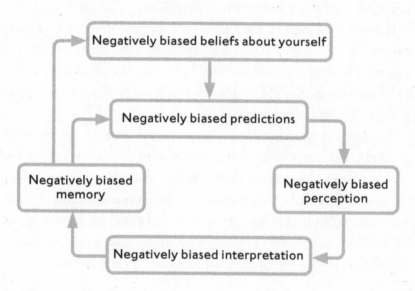

These consistent biases in thinking prevent you from seeing clearly and thus stop you from realising that your Bottom Line is an opinion, not a fact – a kind of prejudice against yourself. They keep your negative views in place, make you anxious and unhappy, restrict your life and prevent you from finding a fairer, more balanced and more accurate perspective on yourself.

What are your Rules for Living?

Even if you believe yourself to be incompetent or inadequate, unattractive or unlovable, you still have to get on with life. Rules for Living help you to do this. They allow you to feel reasonably comfortable with yourself, so long as you obey them. But obeying them is not a choice: you simply have to do it in order to feel OK about yourself, no matter what the cost. And if you fail to do so, then up pops the Bottom Line.

However, Rules also help to keep the Bottom Line in place and so maintain low self-esteem. Let's think back to the people whose stories were told earlier and see how their Bottom Lines fit with their Rules for Living. How do they think they should behave, assuming their central ideas about themselves to be true?

Because they believe their Bottom Lines are true, each of these people has developed Rules for Living to help them get by. For example, Briony believed she was bad – and therefore deserved to be treated badly. So, she decided not to have close relationships, in order to avoid the possibility of being hurt.

To some extent, Rules for Living work. For example, Rajiv's high standards and fear of failure motivated him to perform very well and enabled him to be very successful in his career. But he paid a price for this. His Rules for Living created an increasing sense of strain and made it impossible for him to relax and enjoy his achievements. In addition, his need to perform well meant that work dominated his life, at the expense of personal relationships and leisure time.

	Bottom Line		Rules for Living
Briony	'I am bad'	↑	'If I allow anyone to get close to me, they will hurt and exploit me.'
Rajiv	'I am not good enough'	↑	'Unless I always get it right, I will never get anywhere in life.'
Evie	'I am fat and ugly'	↑	'My worth depends on how I look and what I weigh.'
Jack	'I am unacceptable'	↑	'I must always keep myself under tight control.'
Aaron	'I am worthless'	↑	'No matter what I do, no one will accept me.'
Kate	'I am unlovable'	↑	'Unless I do everything people expect of me, I will be rejected.'
Lin	'I am not important'	↑	'If someone is not interested in me, it is because I am unworthy of interest.'
Chris	'I am stupid'	↑	'It's better not to try than to fail.'
Mike	'I am pathetic'	↑	'I should be able to cope with anything life throws at me.'
Mary	'I am useless'	↑	'My worth depends on caring for other people.'

- What are your Rules for Living? (You may have two or three so extra pages have been provided at the back of the handbook.)

_____

_____

_____

_____

_____

_____

- Think about your Rules and write down how each one helps you in life.

_____

_____

_____

_____

_____

_____

_____

- Now write down how each Rule restricts you in your life.

_____

_____

_____

_____

_____

_____

_____

_____

In Part Three, you will find more details about Rules for Living, their impact on your thoughts and feelings and how you manage your life, and how to change them and liberate yourself from the demands they place upon you.

SUMMARY

1. Your negative beliefs about yourself (your Bottom Line) are opinions, not facts.
2. They are conclusions about yourself based on experience (usually, but not necessarily, early experience). Many different experiences (e.g. abuse, hardship, lack of interest or absence of affection) can contribute to them.
3. Once in place, the Bottom Line can be hard to change. This is because it is supported and strengthened by biased thinking. Biased thinking emphasises experiences that support the Bottom Line, while ignoring experiences that contradict it.
4. The Bottom Line leads you to develop Rules for Living (guidelines which you think you must obey in order to feel comfortable with yourself). These are designed to help you get through life. But in fact, they keep your Bottom Line in place and maintain low self-esteem.

SECTION 3:

What Keeps
Low Self-Esteem Going?

This section will help you to understand:

- what situations trigger your Bottom Line and lead you down anxious or depressed paths
- what anxious predictions are
- the effect of anxious predictions on your feelings and what you do
- how you get the feeling that your Bottom Line has been confirmed and is indeed true
- how self-critical thoughts affect you
- how to draw your own vicious circles, investigating what keeps your low self-esteem going

In this section, we will look at the vicious circles that are triggered when you find yourself in a situation in which you fear that you *might* have broken your Rules for Living or believe that you *have* done so. These are the situations that will activate your Bottom Line.

As we have seen, Rules for Living help to keep low self-esteem at bay in the short term. However, in the long term, they actually keep it going because they make impossible demands – such as perfection, endless approval from others, or complete control over yourself or your world. Because your well-being depends on following these

Rules, it becomes very fragile. If you find yourself in danger of breaking the Rules (e.g. there is a risk of being disliked or of losing control), or believe that you have done so (e.g. someone *did* dislike you, you *did* lose control), then the Bottom Line, which your Rules have protected you against, may rear its ugly head. Then you will begin to feel anxious, insecure or (if you are convinced your Rules *have* been broken) depressed. This process is shown in the flowchart below. This may look a bit complicated, but don't worry. We shall go through it step by step, showing how it works in practice.

The vicious circle that keeps low self-esteem going

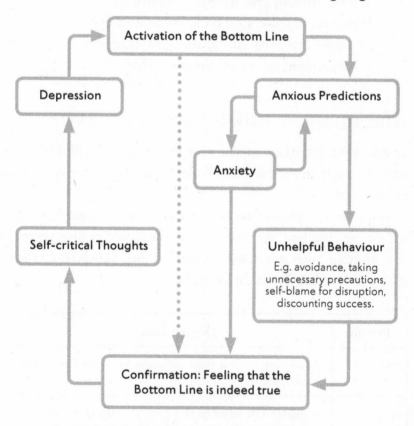

You may find it helpful to start drafting your own vicious circle as you go along, either on paper or electronically. You will find some 'fill in the blanks' sheets at the end of the book and these are also available for download at www.overcoming.co.uk. Here is an opportunity to deepen your understanding of how low self-esteem affects you in everyday life. Keep asking yourself:

- How does this fit with my experience?
- What situations trigger my Bottom Line?
- How do my anxious predictions affect my emotions and my body state?
- What do I do (or not do) to stop them coming true?
- How do I feel when I think they have come true, and it seems as if my Bottom Line has been confirmed?
- What sort of self-critical thoughts do I have?
- How do these self-critical thoughts affect my feelings, my behaviour and my beliefs about myself?

What situations activate your Bottom Line?

Exactly what situations trigger your Bottom Line will depend on what it is, and on the particular Rules for Living you have adopted to cope with it.

Think back to the people you met when we discussed how low self-esteem develops. As you will see, the situations that triggered their Bottom Lines were closely linked to their beliefs about themselves, and to their Rules for Living:

Person	Trigger situations
Briony:	Fearing that her true (bad) self might be revealed and people would hurt her
Rajiv:	Feeling that he might be unable to meet the high standards he had set himself, or being criticised by someone else

Evie:	Noticing that she had gained weight, or needing to buy clothes and fearing that she might attract stares or not fit into the size she thought she should be
Jack:	Feeling very energetic or emotional, or being disapproved of
Aaron:	Feeling vulnerable to attack or rejection, including in close relationships
Kate:	Being unable to do what was expected of her, or having to ask for help
Lin:	Showing her work in public
Chris:	Having to write, especially if he had to do it in front of other people, or having to face any challenge (especially any intellectual challenge)
Mike:	Noticing signs that he was still upset and not his normal self
Mary:	Seeing someone who needed help and support she was no longer able to give

So, the situations that activate your Bottom Line are those in which you think the Rules *might* be broken (there is an element of uncertainty) or definitely *have* been broken (you are quite sure). These situations cast doubt on your sense of your own worth. They may be quite big events (e.g. losing a job, having a serious illness, a relationship breaking up). Or they may be little everyday 'ups and downs' that you barely even notice. In order to understand what keeps your poor opinion of yourself going, you need to learn to recognise the changes in how you feel that tell you that your Bottom Line has been activated, and to observe closely the feelings, thoughts and behaviour that follow.

Think back over the last week:

1. Note down any situations when you felt anxious, uncomfortable, depressed, or doubtful about your ability to handle what was going on.

_____

_____

_____

_____

_____

_____

2. Note down any situations when you suspected that you were not making the impression you wanted to make.

_____

_____

_____

_____

_____

_____

3. Note down any situations when you felt that things were getting on top of you.

_____

_____

_____

_____

_____

_____

4. Do you notice any similarities between these situations?

_____

_____

_____

_____

_____

_____

5. If so, what do they tell you about your own personal Rules for Living? What do you have to do or be in order to feel OK about yourself?

_____

_____

_____

_____

_____

_____

6. What Rules did you think you were breaking, or in danger of breaking?

_____

_____

_____

_____

_____

_____

7. What ideas about yourself came into your mind at these times?

_____

_____

_____

_____

_____

8. Did you use any unkind or critical words to describe yourself? What were they? They may reflect your central negative beliefs about yourself (your Bottom Line).

_____

_____

_____

_____

_____

_____

When the Rules might be broken: the anxious path

Anxious predictions

When you are in a trigger situation that activates your Bottom Line because you fear your Rules *might* be broken, you start to worry about what may happen. These worries are your anxious predictions.

For example, imagine that you have to give a talk to a group of people – perhaps to colleagues at work, students in a class, or members of your church. Most people find this kind of situation rather anxiety-provoking. What is *your* immediate reaction when you imagine having to stand up and speak to a group of people? Tick the answer/s that most closely match what you predict would happen:

1. What thoughts come to mind?

    ☐ a. 'I couldn't do it.'
    ☐ b. 'I'd make a total fool of myself.'
    ☐ c. 'No one would want to listen to me.'
    ☐ d. 'I'd get so anxious I would have to run out.'

2. How do you imagine the audience reacting?

    ☐ a. 'They would probably be bored.'
    ☐ b. 'They would think I was weird.'
    ☐ c. 'They might sit there smiling kindly, but secretly they'd be thinking what a sad case I was.'
    ☐ d. 'They would be disappointed because I wouldn't live up to their expectations.'

3. How do you imagine yourself reacting physically?

    ☐ a. 'I'd go red in the face.'
    ☐ b. 'My hands would feel sweaty.'

☐ c. 'My mouth would probably go dry.'
☐ d. 'My heart would be racing.'
☐ e. 'All the muscles in my face would tense up.'
☐ f. 'I'd have butterflies in my stomach.'
☐ g. 'My mind would go blank.'

In challenging situations, a person with low self-esteem naturally assumes that the worst will happen – they get caught up in making anxious predictions. Naturally these make them frightened, with all the physical symptoms that go with that. These 'symptoms' may then feed into even more anxious predictions – what if they can't complete the talk, or go blank, or start shaking uncontrollably? What on earth will everyone think? All this of course adds to the stress of the situation.

How do anxious predictions impact on your behaviour?
Anxious predictions may lead you to:

1. **Avoid challenging situations**
2. **Take unnecessary precautions**
3. **Place too much weight on minor disruptions in your performance**
4. **Discount success**

Unhelpful behaviour

1 Avoiding challenging situations

If you believe your anxious predictions that the worst will happen, it makes sense to do whatever you can to stop this from occurring. You might decide to avoid the situation altogether. For instance, you might phone the person who had asked you to give the talk and tell them you had flu and would not be able to make it. Or you might simply not turn up.

How would you avoid giving a talk to a group? What excuses would you make?

_____

_____

_____

_____

_____

_____

No doubt in the short term you would feel better if you avoided the situation (what a relief, you got out of it). But unfortunately, avoiding the situation would prevent you from finding out for yourself whether or not your anxious predictions were in fact correct. Things might actually have gone much better than you predicted.

So, in order to develop your confidence in yourself and improve your self-esteem, you need to begin approaching situations that you have been avoiding. Otherwise you will never gain the information you need in order to have a realistic, balanced and kinder view of yourself.

2 Taking unnecessary precautions

Rather than avoiding the situation altogether, you might decide to give your talk, but take lots of precautions in order to ensure that your worst fears did not come true and avoid bruising your self-esteem. For example, you might spend much longer than necessary rehearsing your talk so as to be sure you got it right in every detail.

Or you might avoid making eye contact with the audience, in case you saw them looking bored. Or you might leave no time for questions at the end – in case you were unable to answer them.

If you had to give a talk, what precautions would you take – in order to ensure that your worst fears were not realised?

_____

_____

_____

_____

_____

_____

The problem with taking precautions is that (like avoidance) they prevent you from finding out whether your fears are actually true, or not. Instead, you are left with the sense that you had a narrow escape, a near miss – your success (and so your feeling of self-worth) was entirely due to the precautions you took. Again, an opportunity to learn from experience that things do not necessarily turn out as badly as we predict, and perhaps to begin to update your Bottom Line and your Rules, has been missed.

So, in order to become more confident, you will need to approach challenging situations without taking precautions. This is the only way to discover that your precautions are unnecessary – you can get what you want out of life and be the kind of person you want to be, without them.

3 Placing too much weight on minor disruptions in your performance

Sometimes performance is genuinely disrupted by anxiety. While giving your talk, for example, you might find yourself stammering, your notes might shake in your hand, or your mind might go blank. These things happen, even to experienced speakers.

If your performance was disrupted by anxiety, what would your reaction be? What thoughts might come into your mind?

_____

_____

_____

_____

_____

_____

Self-confident people might notice these signs of anxiety and simply see them as an understandable reaction to being under pressure. They might believe that being nervous under these circumstances was quite normal and be pretty sure that their anxiety was much less obvious to other people than it was to them. As far as confident people are concerned, being anxious does not matter particularly. They can accept a less than perfect performance, and they would not see it as reflecting on their worth as people. If you have low self-esteem, however, then you will probably see any difficulties as evidence of your usual uselessness or incompetence or whatever. That is, they say something about you *as a person*.

So, to feel happier with yourself, you will need to start viewing your weaknesses simply as aspects of being a normal, imperfect human being, rather than reasons to condemn yourself out of hand.

4 Discounting success

Despite your anxieties, your talk might in fact go just fine. Perhaps you said what you wanted to say, people seemed interested, you didn't get too nervous, there were some interesting questions, and you answered them well.

If this happened to you, would you give yourself a pat on the back? Or would you have a sneaking suspicion that you had done it by the skin of your teeth: the audience was just being kind, or you were lucky – it was probably a one-off?

How would you react if your talk went well? What kind of thoughts would come to mind?

_____

_____

_____

_____

_____

_____

_____

_____

Even when things go well, low self-esteem can remove your pleasure in what you achieve and make you likely to ignore or discount anything that does not fit your negative view of yourself (remember the negative biases in thinking that we described earlier on).

So, learning to notice and take pleasure in your achievements and in the good things in your life is part of developing healthy self-esteem. Part Two of the handbook will focus in detail on how to do this.

How is your Bottom Line confirmed?

Whether you avoid challenging situations altogether, hedge them about with unnecessary precautions, condemn yourself if they do not go well, or discount and deny how well they actually did go, you are likely to end up in the same place. That is, you will almost certainly end up feeling that your negative self-beliefs have been confirmed – they are indeed true. You may actually say this to yourself in so many words: 'There you are, I always knew it, I really *am* . . . ' Or you may just feel sad or gloomy or see an image in your mind's eye of yourself looking stupid or awkward or whatever, or perhaps have a sinking feeling in your stomach or notice that your neck and shoulders have tensed up. Whatever form your sense of confirmation takes, the essential message is that what you always knew about yourself has been proved right, yet again. This opens the door to self-critical thinking.

How do self-critical thoughts affect you?

At this point, the feel of things shifts from anxious to something heavier, gloomier. Once you believe that your negative ideas about yourself have been confirmed, you may well react by criticising and condemning yourself as a person. Self-critical thoughts may just flash briefly through your mind – or you may get trapped in a spiral of vicious attacks on yourself. Just as anxious predictions can shade into extended worries, so self-critical thoughts can easily shade into rumination – preoccupation with how far you have fallen short of your standards and what that says about you. These may have a hopeless feel to them. What else can you expect? You'll always be like this, and that's all there is to it.

Here is what Rajiv (the boy whose father quizzed him at the supper table) said to himself when his computer crashed, and he lost an important document he was rushing to complete:

'Now look what you've done. You are a complete idiot. How could you be so stupid? You always mess things up – absolutely typical. You'll never amount to anything – you simply haven't got what it takes. Why are you always so useless?'

The computer crash wasn't actually Rajiv's fault at all, but he still believed that it confirmed his negative ideas about himself. This made him angry and frustrated, and made it extremely difficult for him to calm down and work out how to solve the problem. It also made him think that he would always fail at everything in his life. And then naturally his mood dropped, and he began to feel depressed. And all this had an impact on his behaviour. He had been due to go away at the weekend with some friends, but he couldn't face it. He sat around at home doing nothing in particular, brooding about the future. He couldn't see any real chance that things would ever change, so what was the point of carrying on? These understandable reactions then tapped into further self-critical thinking. Why couldn't he pull himself together and get on with it? And his mood dipped even further.

Self-critical thoughts, like anxious predictions, have a major impact on how we feel and how we deal with our lives. They help to keep low self-esteem going. Think about your own reactions when things do not work out as you planned:

- What runs through your mind in these situations?
- Are you hard on yourself?
- Do you put yourself down and call yourself names, like Rajiv?
- How do you feel at these times?
- What impact does self-criticism have on your behaviour? Do you notice things you then do – or stop doing – that tend to reinforce your self-critical thoughts (e.g. isolating yourself, not taking care of yourself properly, dropping out of your normal routine)?

- Does self-criticism make it easier, or harder, for you to solve problems and tackle difficulties?

Being critical of yourself, especially if you believe that what you criticise in yourself cannot be changed, can pull you down into depression. This may be only a brief sadness, quickly banished by spending time with people you care about, or by engaging in an absorbing activity. Or it may develop into a longer-term condition, especially if you have suffered from serious depression in the past. If this is the case for you, you may need to work on the depression in its own right before you begin to tackle low self-esteem (see p. 5 for information on how to recognise depression that might need treatment).

Whether it is brief or longer-term, depression completes the vicious circle. Once you become depressed, depressed mood in itself makes you more self-critical and more likely to see the future in a gloomy light. So, depression keeps the Bottom Line activated, and encourages you to predict the worst. Bingo! You have a circular process that may continue, if you do not interrupt it, for long periods of time.

On the page overleaf is the vicious circle Rajiv drew up after his computer crashed.

Rajiv's vicious circle

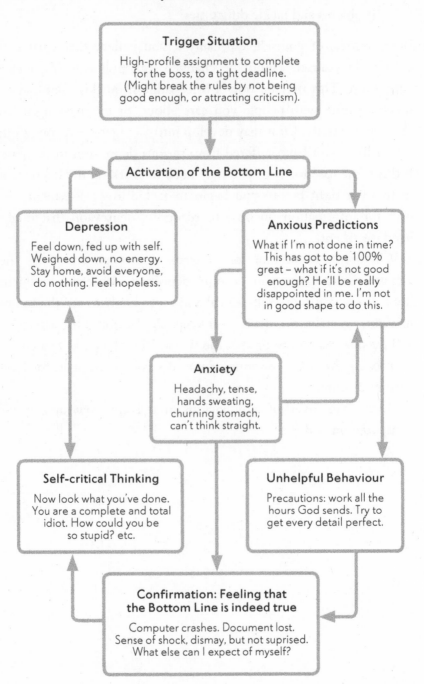

Trigger Situation

High-profile assignment to complete for the boss, to a tight deadline. (Might break the rules by not being good enough, or attracting criticism).

Activation of the Bottom Line

Depression

Feel down, fed up with self. Weighed down, no energy. Stay home, avoid everyone, do nothing. Feel hopeless.

Anxious Predictions

What if I'm not done in time? This has got to be 100% great – what if it's not good enough? He'll be really disappointed in me. I'm not in good shape to do this.

Anxiety

Headachy, tense, hands sweating, churning stomach, can't think straight.

Self-critical Thinking

Now look what you've done. You are a complete and total idiot. How could you be so stupid? etc.

Unhelpful Behaviour

Precautions: work all the hours God sends. Try to get every detail perfect.

Confirmation: Feeling that the Bottom Line is indeed true

Computer crashes. Document lost. Sense of shock, dismay, but not suprised. What else can I expect of myself?

When the Rules definitely have been broken: the depressed path

When a person with low self-esteem believes that the Rules definitely *have* been broken, then rather than following the anxious path described above, he or she may immediately experience the sense that the Bottom Line has been confirmed – there is simply no doubt that it is true. In this case, there may be a short cut directly from activation to confirmation of the Bottom Line (see below), moving straight into self-criticism, depression, hopelessness and self-defeating behaviour, rather than experiencing the uncertainty reflected in the anxious path. This mini-vicious circle can then cycle on, as we saw with Rajiv, keeping the person trapped in a low mood.

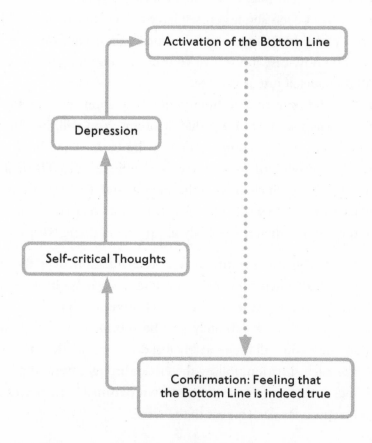

Rajiv experienced this on another occasion at work. His boss made a passing remark about an error he had made on an assignment. Rajiv's instant response was to see the remark as confirmation that he was indeed not good enough (his Bottom Line). Once again, he began to berate himself and his mood dipped. He forced himself to keep going to work but felt dreadful for several days and even considered resigning.

How to draw your own vicious circle

As you have read through this part of the handbook, you have been asked to consider how you personally might react in particular situations, to reflect on your own anxious predictions and their impact on your emotional state and your behaviour, your own sense that your negative beliefs about yourself have been confirmed, your own typical self-critical thoughts, and the impact these have on how you feel, and on how easy it is to live your life as you wish and to accept and value yourself just as you are.

Now is the time to fine-tune your observations by drawing up your own vicious circles in real-life situations. You will find 'blanks' over the page, and additional blanks at the back of the book, and available for download from www.overcoming.co.uk. These show the headings for each element of the anxious and depressed paths and leave space for you to write. Here is a chance for you to find out more about the system when it is actually in operation, doing what it does.

- See if you can identify at least one situation over the next few days when you feel your Rules *might* be broken (you will know because you will feel anxious), and one when you believe they definitely *have* been broken (you will know because you will immediately feel down, rather than anxious).
- For each situation, follow the circle through, using the headings as a prompt to note your own personal experiences and reactions for each aspect of the circle.

- The exact flavour of the sequence is different from person to person, and indeed from situation to situation. So, try to capture as precisely as you can your own anxious predictions (word for word, or perhaps images in your mind's eye), how you personally experience anxiety, what the sense of confirmation feels like for you, how you criticise yourself, how low mood affects you, and so on.
- Aim to record what you notice as soon as possible after it happens, so that it is still clear in your mind.
- If you wish, when you have completed one circle, you can repeat the process using a different trigger situation. Your task is to get curious about what keeps low self-esteem going – to be your own detective and ferret it all out. Mapping out more than one circle will help you to begin to notice old habits – repeated patterns in your thoughts, your feelings and body sensations, and what you do.

Anxious vicious circle

Trigger Situation

Situation where you fear your Rule *might* be broken

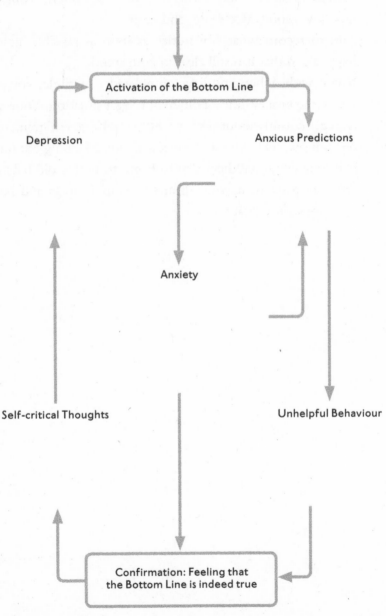

Activation of the Bottom Line

Depression

Anxious Predictions

Anxiety

Self-critical Thoughts

Unhelpful Behaviour

Confirmation: Feeling that
the Bottom Line is indeed true

Depressed vicious circle

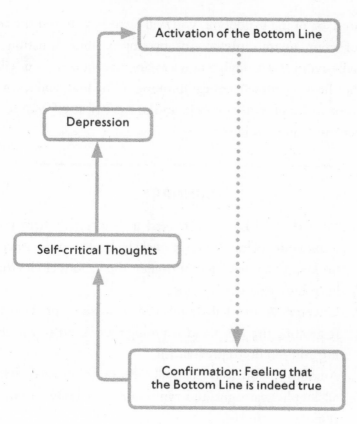

Drawing your own vicious circles will increase your awareness of how your patterns of anxious and self-critical thinking operate to keep low self-esteem going. This is your first step towards breaking the circle and moving on.

Breaking the vicious circle

In Part Two of the handbook, you will learn how to test the accuracy of your anxious predictions by approaching situations you normally avoid and dropping unnecessary precautions. You will also find out how to nip self-critical thinking in the bud, and learn how to accept and appreciate yourself, and to treat yourself with respect, consideration and kindness.

SUMMARY

1. Your Bottom Line is activated in situations where you think your Rules for Living *might* be broken or *have* been broken. Once activated, it triggers the vicious circles that keep low self-esteem going.
2. Uncertainty and self-doubt lead to anxious predictions (expecting the worst and assuming there is little or nothing you can do to prevent it).
3. Anxious predictions naturally produce anxiety, with all its physical signs and symptoms (the body's normal response to threat).
4. They also affect your behaviour, leading you to complete avoidance, taking unnecessary precautions, or placing too much weight on minor disruptions in performance. Even if things go well, your prejudice against yourself will make it difficult for you to recognise or accept this.
5. The end result is a feeling that your Bottom Line has been confirmed; it is indeed true.
6. Confirmation then triggers self-critical thinking.
7. Self-critical thinking often leads to a dip in mood, which may develop into a full-scale depression.
8. Low mood continues to activate your Bottom Line, thus completing the vicious circle.

THOUGHTS AND REFLECTIONS

THOUGHTS AND REFLECTIONS

PART TWO:

Checking Out Anxious Predictions, Questioning Self-Critical Thoughts and Enhancing Self-Acceptance

Introduction

So far, we have focused on understanding how low self-esteem works – how it develops, and the thinking habits and unhelpful patterns of behaviour that keep it going (the vicious circle). Now you will be able to use this understanding as a basis for undermining old, negative beliefs about yourself and beginning instead to cultivate healthy self-esteem.

The first step is to tackle the predictions that make you anxious in situations where you fear that your Rules for Living *might* be broken. This means exploring three core skills:

1. **Awareness** Closely observing and recording what happens.

2. **Re-thinking** Learning to step back from your unhelpful thoughts and question them, rather than simply accepting them as accurate and true.

3. **Experiments** Using direct experience as a way of checking out old perspectives and discovering whether new ones will genuinely be more helpful to you.

These core skills are central to your journey towards a new, kinder and more balanced view of yourself. So, this part of the handbook lays a strong foundation on which you will be able to build. You will find that the same core skills will come into play when dealing with self-critical thinking, learning to recognise your good qualities and treating yourself with respect and consideration, developing less harshly demanding Rules for Living, and creating a new Bottom Line.

SECTION 1:

Checking Out
Anxious Predictions

This section will help you to understand:

- why we make predictions
- how anxious predictions keep low self-esteem going
- what anxious predictions are
- how to spot your own anxious predictions and the unnecessary precautions that you take to stop them from coming true
- how to find alternatives to your anxious predictions
- how to check out your anxious predictions in practice
- how to use what you discover to come up with new, more accurate and helpful predictions and work out what to do next

Why do we make predictions?

We all make predictions (e.g. 'If I press this switch, the light will come on', 'If I stand in the rain, I will get wet') and then act on them. Many of these are so well practised and automatic that we do not even notice them – we just act as if they were true. We use information from our experience to confirm our predictions or to change them. Acting in line with predictions is generally a useful strategy, as long as we keep an open mind and are willing to change our thinking in the light of new information.

The problem with low self-esteem of course is that it makes it hard to do this. Predictions seem like statements of fact, rather than hunches or guesses that may or may not be accurate. In this section, you will learn how to recognise anxious predictions, how to question them and look for more realistic perspectives, and how to check them out in practice. In this way you will free up real choices for yourself in how you lead your life, rather than always feeling obliged to tread a narrow path.

Imagine that you're about to start a new job. Look at the following predictions and write 'A' next to the ones that sound anxious and 'R' next to the ones that sound realistic:

a. 'My colleagues will probably be helpful.' _____

b. 'I'm bound to get everything wrong.' _____

c. 'I just know I won't be able to cope with the pressure.' _____

d. 'I may find the work hard at first, but I'll soon get the hang of it.' _____

e. 'My colleagues will think I'm stupid and laugh at me behind my back.' _____

f. 'If I make a mistake, they'll all think I'm an idiot for evermore.'

_____

g. 'I will be nervous on my first day, but everyone gets nervous when they start a new job.' _____

h. 'If I make a silly mistake, people will probably tease me a bit and then forget about it.' _____

Anxious predictions: b, c, e, f
Realistic predictions: a, d, g, h

IT'S WORTH REMEMBERING . . .

If you have low self-esteem, you will probably treat your anxious predictions as facts, rather than ideas which may or may not turn out to be true. This makes it difficult to stand back and look at the evidence objectively.

The vicious circle we mapped out in Part One, and which is repeated on the next page, shows how you are likely to make anxious predictions in situations where your **Bottom Line** (e.g. 'I'm stupid' or 'I'm unlovable') has been activated and you think there is a risk that one or more of your personal **Rules for Living** *might* be broken – you are not sure, but it could happen. This is the anxious path highlighted on the right-hand side of the vicious circle shown below.

Think back to the people you met in Part One. If, for example, like Chris, your Bottom Line was 'I'm stupid', your main Rule for Living might be 'It's better not to try than to fail.' The system would be activated by situations where there was a danger that you *might* fail. Whereas if, like Kate, your Bottom Line was 'I'm unlovable', your main Rule for Living might be 'Unless I do everything people expect of me, I will be rejected.' In this case, the system would be activated by situations where you feared you *might* not be able to meet others' expectations.

How anxious predictions keep low self-esteem going

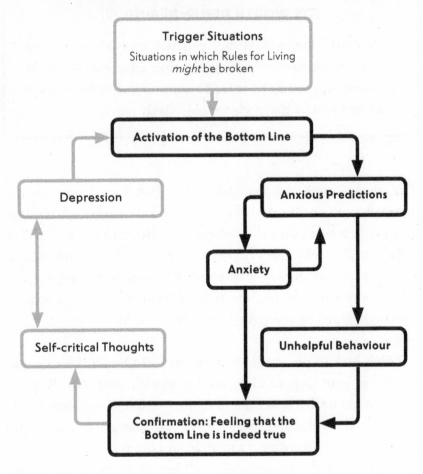

Doubt and uncertainty will lead you to wonder what is going to happen next (e.g. 'Will I be able to cope?' 'Will people like me?'). The answers to these questions – which are really predictions about what *might* go wrong – spark anxiety and lead you to take a whole range of precautions to prevent the worst from happening. Unfortunately, in the long run, these precautions rarely work. You just end up feeling that your Bottom Line has been confirmed yet again or, at best, that you have had a narrow escape.

What are anxious predictions?

So, we make anxious predictions when we fear that we are about to break Rules that are important to our sense of self-esteem.

ANXIOUS PREDICTIONS

These predictions usually involve:

1. **Overestimating the chances that something bad will happen**
2. **Overestimating how bad it will be if something bad does happen**
3. **Underestimating our ability to deal with the worst, if it happens**
4. **Underestimating outside factors, such as other people's support**

Let's take Kate, who we met in Part One (p. 33), as an example to illustrate these different types of anxious predictions. You may recall that she was brought up by elderly middle-class parents who tried their best to give their daughter a sound start in life. But they had difficulty showing her open affection (kisses, cuddles, pet names), and could only show their love by practical means – very different from what she saw in other families. You may recall that Kate concluded this must be a reflection of something wrong with her – her Bottom Line was that she was unlovable. Her Rules for Living were that if she failed to meet others' expectations she would be rejected. And asking for what she needed would only lead to disappointment.

1. Overestimating the chances that something bad will happen

Kate worked in a hairdresser's. She and her workmates took it in turns to go out and buy the lunchtime sandwiches. One day, when it was her turn, her boss forgot to pay her back for his sandwich. Kate felt completely unable to ask for what she was owed. She was convinced that, if she did so, her boss would despise her and think she was mean. This was despite the fact that she knew from months of working for him that he was a kind, thoughtful man who cared about his employees' welfare. She took no account of the evidence, which suggested that in fact he was likely to be embarrassed, apologise and immediately give her what she was entitled to.

In just the same way, in a situation where you think it will be hard to stick to your Rules for Living, you may get over-anxious that something will go wrong. Think back to a time when you overestimated the chances that something bad would happen.

When and where did it happen?

_____

_____

_____

_____

What exactly did you think would happen (what was your prediction)?

_____

_____

_____

_____

2 Overestimating how bad it will be if something bad does happen

When Kate looked into the future, she could not see her boss being mildly inconvenienced by having to pay her back, and then quickly forgetting all about it. She assumed that asking for what he owed her would permanently change their relationship. He would never look at her in the same way again, and she would probably need to find another job – which would be difficult, because he would not want to give her a reference. Then she would have to go back to her parents' house and live on state benefits and would be completely stuck. Kate could clearly see all this happening, in her mind's eye.

At the heart of anxious predictions is the idea that the worst possible thing will happen and that, when it does, it won't be over quickly. Instead it will be a huge personal disaster. So your turn now to think back to a time when you overestimated how bad it would be if something bad did happen.

When and where did it happen?

_____

_____

_____

_____

What was your prediction about how bad things would be?

_____

_____

_____

_____

3 Underestimating your ability to deal with the worst, if it does happen

Kate assumed that, no matter what she did, her boss would reject her. It did not occur to her that she could stand up to him, if he did indeed respond as she predicted, and remind him assertively that she was entitled to get her money back. Nor did she take account of her professional skill and experience, which in fact made it very likely that she would find other employment quite easily.

When people are anxious, they are apt to think that, if the worst does happen, there will be nothing they can do to prevent it or make it manageable. Think back to a time when you underestimated your ability to deal with the worst.

When and where did it happen?

_____

_____

_____

_____

What was your prediction about how you would cope?

_____

_____

_____

_____

4 Underestimating outside resources such as other people's support

Kate completely overlooked the support she would get from her workmates, friends and family if her boss reacted so unreasonably.

Anxiety may lead you to underestimate things outside yourself that might improve the situation. Think back to a time when you underestimated such resources.

When and where did it happen?

_____

_____

_____

_____

What was your prediction about what outside resources might be there to help you?

_____

_____

_____

_____

How to spot your anxious predictions and the unnecessary precautions you take (Core skill 1: Awareness)

Anxious predictions give you a strong sense that you are at risk – of failure, of rejection, of losing control, of making a fool of yourself. So, like any sensible person facing a threat, you take precautions to stop the worst from happening. These may help you to feel better in the short term, but unfortunately, they stop you from finding out through direct experience whether your anxious predictions have any basis in reality. And so, in the long run, they help to keep your low self-esteem going.

In order to get a more realistic view of what is likely to happen in situations you fear, you first of all need to become fully aware of your anxious predictions and the unnecessary precautions you take. The best way to do this is to keep a record for a few days, by hand or electronically, noticing what is running through your mind as soon as the anxiety starts, and spotting what you do to protect yourself. Keeping a record will help you to fine-tune your observational skills, and you may also find that seeing your thoughts written down helps you to stand back from them a bit, instead of having them trapped inside your head. The chart filled in by Kate, on p. 93, illustrates how to go about it.

You will find other Predictions and Precautions Charts for you to fill in on pp. 94–100, and further guidelines to help you complete the charts on pp. 101–104. There are more at the end of the book, and you can also download them from www.overcoming.co.uk.

Predictions and Precautions Chart: Kate

Date/Time	Situation What were you doing when you began to feel anxious?	Emotions and body sensations (e.g. anxious, panicky, tense, heart racing). Rate 0–100 for intensity.	Anxious predictions What exactly was going through your mind when you began to feel anxious (e.g. thoughts in words, images)? Rate each one 0–100% for how far you believed it.	Precautions What did you do to stop your predictions coming true (e.g. avoid the situation, take precautions)?
6 February	Bought sandwich for Ian for lunch. He forgot to pay me back.	Anxious 85 Embarrassed 80 Heart racing 90 Sweaty 70 Hot 90	If I ask for the money, he will think I'm really mean 90% It will spoil our relationship forever 80% I will have to find another job 70% I won't be able to 70% I'll be stuck at home with no money 70%	Avoid him altogether If I did ask, I would: • be very apologetic • not look at him directly • keep my voice down • tell him it didn't really matter • get it over and done with as fast as possible and then run away

Predictions and Precautions Chart

Date/Time	Situation What were you doing when you began to feel anxious?	Emotions and body sensations (e.g. anxious, panicky, tense, heart racing). Rate 0–100 for intensity.	Anxious predictions What exactly was going through your mind when you began to feel anxious (e.g. thoughts in words, images)? Rate each one 0–100% for how far you believed it.	Precautions What did you do to stop your predictions coming true (e.g. avoid the situation, take precautions)?

Predictions and Precautions Chart

Date/Time	Situation What were you doing when you began to feel anxious?	Emotions and body sensations (e.g. anxious, panicky, tense, heart racing). Rate 0–100 for intensity.	Anxious predictions What exactly was going through your mind when you began to feel anxious (e.g. thoughts in words, images)? Rate each one 0–100% for how far you believed it.	Precautions What did you do to stop your predictions coming true (e.g. avoid the situation, take precautions)?

Predictions and Precautions Chart

Date/Time	Situation What were you doing when you began to feel anxious?	Emotions and body sensations (e.g. anxious, panicky, tense, heart racing). Rate 0–100 for intensity.	Anxious predictions What exactly was going through your mind when you began to feel anxious (e.g. thoughts in words, images)? Rate each one 0–100% for how far you believed it.	Precautions What did you do to stop your predictions coming true (e.g. avoid the situation, take precautions)?

Predictions and Precautions Chart

| Date/Time | Situation
What were you doing when you began to feel anxious? | Emotions and body sensations
(e.g. anxious, panicky, tense, heart racing).
Rate 0–100 for intensity. | Anxious predictions
What exactly was going through your mind when you began to feel anxious (e.g. thoughts in words, images)? Rate each one 0–100% for how far you believed it. | Precautions
What did you do to stop your predictions coming true (e.g. avoid the situation, take precautions)? |
|---|---|---|---|---|
| | | | | |

Predictions and Precautions Chart

Date/Time	Situation What were you doing when you began to feel anxious?	Emotions and body sensations (e.g. anxious, panicky, tense, heart racing). Rate 0–100 for intensity.	Anxious predictions What exactly was going through your mind when you began to feel anxious (e.g. thoughts in words, images)? Rate each one 0–100% for how far you believed it.	Precautions What did you do to stop your predictions coming true (e.g. avoid the situation, take precautions)?

Predictions and Precautions Chart

Date/Time	Situation What were you doing when you began to feel anxious?	Emotions and body sensations (e.g. anxious, panicky, tense, heart racing). Rate 0–100 for intensity.	Anxious predictions What exactly was going through your mind when you began to feel anxious (e.g. thoughts in words, images)? Rate each one 0–100% for how far you believed it.	Precautions What did you do to stop your predictions coming true (e.g. avoid the situation, take precautions)?

Predictions and Precautions Chart

Date/Time	Situation What were you doing when you began to feel anxious?	Emotions and body sensations (e.g. anxious, panicky, tense, heart racing). Rate 0–100 for intensity.	Anxious predictions What exactly was going through your mind when you began to feel anxious (e.g. thoughts in words, images)? Rate each one 0–100% for how far you believed it.	Precautions What did you do to stop your predictions coming true (e.g. avoid the situation, take precautions)?

The information you gather by keeping a careful record will put you in a good position to begin to question your predictions and check them out by doing the things you are afraid of without taking unnecessary precautions. This is how you will begin to gain confidence and boost your self-esteem.

See if you can bring a spirit of interest and curiosity to your investigations. Just exactly how does this intriguing mind of yours work? Day by day, you may begin to notice patterns emerging, old automatic habits of thought coming up again and again. Once you can see them clearly, the process of re-thinking them can begin.

If at all possible, make your record at the time when you actually experience the anxiety. If this is not possible, make a careful mental note of what happens and complete your record as soon as you can. It is often difficult to tune in to anxious predictions when you are no longer feeling anxious. They can flash through your mind so quickly that afterwards it is difficult to remember what they were, especially if they took the form of images rather than words. Or they may seem ridiculous or exaggerated when you are not in the situation, and so it may be difficult to accept how convincing they were and how anxious you felt at the time. Here are some guidelines to help you fill in each section.

Date/time

- When exactly did you begin to feel anxious?
- Can you see a pattern? For instance, do you tend to get anxious on weekdays at work, or at the weekends when you are expected to socialise?

The situation

- What was happening when you started to feel anxious? What were you doing? Where were you? Who were you with? Try to recreate the situation in your mind's eye.

- Or was it that something uncomfortable came to mind – a memory perhaps, or a concern about something in the future?

Your feelings

- What emotions did you feel? Were you anxious, panicky, frightened, pressured, worried, frustrated, irritable, impatient – or what?
- Rate each emotion between 0 and 100, according to how strong it was (100 would mean it was as strong as it could possibly be; 50 would mean it was moderately strong; 5 would mean there was just a hint of emotion, and so on).

Body sensations

- Did you feel your muscles tensing up – for example, in your jaw, forehead, shoulders or hands?
- Did your heart feel as if it was speeding up, pounding heavily or missing a beat?
- Were you holding your breath, breathing faster or breathing unevenly?
- Was it hard to focus on what was going on? Did your mind go blank? Did you feel muddled or confused?
- Did you have problems with your digestion (e.g. churning stomach, 'butterflies', needing to go to the toilet repeatedly)?
- Did you have other physical symptoms (e.g. shakiness; sweating; feeling weak, dizzy or faint; numbness or tingling sensations; blurred or tunnel vision)?
- Make a note of your body sensations, and rate them between 0 and 100 according to how strong they were, just as you rated your emotions.

Your anxious predictions

- What exactly was going through your mind just before you began to feel anxious? And as your anxiety built up?
- What did you think was going to go wrong, or was already going wrong? (Write down your predictions, word for word, just as they occur to you.)
- If your predictions took the form of pictures in your mind's eye (snapshots or freeze frames, or a movie sequence with events following on from one another), briefly describe them.
- Were your predictions in the form of short exclamations, such as 'Oh my God!' or 'Here I go again'? These exclamations are just disguised ways of making anxious predictions. See if you can unpack them. What did you fear was going to happen?
- Or were your predictions in the form of questions, such as 'Will they like me?' If so, look for the prediction hiding behind the question, e.g. 'They won't like me.'
- When you have written down your predictions, rate each one (verbal or visual) between 0 and 100 per cent, according to how strongly you believed it when you were at your most anxious. (100 per cent means you were fully convinced, with no shadow of doubt; 50 means you were in two minds; 5 means you thought there was a remote possibility; and so on.)

Your precautions

- What steps did you take to ensure that your predictions did not come true?
- Did you completely avoid the situation? Or did you enter the situation but take precautions to prevent yourself from breaking your Rules for Living?
- Write down what you did to protect yourself, in as much detail as possible.

Keep your record for a week, filling in one chart per day. By the end of the week, you should have a pretty good idea of the situations in which you feel anxious, the predictions that spark off your anxiety, and the precautions you take to prevent the worst from happening.

How to find alternatives to your anxious predictions (Core skill 2: Re-thinking)

Anxious predictions make you feel bad and encourage you to take precautions that only keep the vicious circle of low self-esteem going. So, finding alternatives to them will help you to feel better, to approach life and enjoy your experiences more confidently, and to feel free to be your true self.

Once you can identify your predictions and precautions as they happen, the next step is to learn to stand back and question your predictions, rather than accepting them as fact. Here is where you begin to practise the second and third of the three core skills we identified in the introduction: re-thinking (questioning your predictions so that you can arrive at more realistic alternatives); and experiments (checking out your new alternatives by approaching – instead of avoiding – the situations you fear and dropping your precautions). This last step probably sounds rather scary, but it is the only way to be sure that your new perspectives are genuinely accurate and helpful. So, let experience be your teacher.

You can use the key questions listed on p. 114 to help you discover more helpful and realistic perspectives and tackle the negative (biased) thinking that contributes to anxiety. Each time you find an alternative to one of your anxious predictions, write it down on the chart on p. 108 and rate how far you believe it (from 0 to 100 per cent). You may well not believe your alternatives fully to begin with, but you should at least be prepared to accept that they might theoretically be true. Once you have a chance to test them out in practice, your degree of belief will increase. When you have found all the alternatives you can think of, move across to the final column on the chart to assess the outcome of what you have done. Now that you have found alternatives to your predictions, how do you feel? And how far do you now believe your original predictions (0–100 per cent)? You may not have stopped believing in them completely. Once again, this is where checking them out in practice will be helpful.

The **Questioning Anxious Predictions Chart** filled in by Kate (p. 106) will give you a sense of how to go about questioning your predictions and finding more realistic and helpful alternatives to them.

You will find blank **Questioning Anxious Predictions Charts** for you to fill in on pp. 108–13. Aim to complete the sheets for at least three days, using one chart per day. This will give you a chance to use these new skills in a range of situations. Feel free to continue beyond three days if you feel it would be helpful – once again, you will find a copy at the end of the book, and you can download them from www.overcoming.co.uk. The best way to develop and fine-tune skills of any kind is to practise them repeatedly and note the results. Of course this takes time, and it is important to give it the time it deserves. The more you do this, the more your confidence in your ability to tackle anxious predictions will grow. You will find further guidelines to help you complete the charts on pp. 114–117.

Questioning Anxious Predictions Chart: Kate

Date/Time	Situation	Emotions and body sensations Rate 0–100% for intensity.	Anxious predictions Rate belief 0–100%	Alternative perspectives Use the key questions to find other views of the situation. Rate belief 0–100%.	Outcome 1. What did you do instead of taking your usual precautions? 2. What were the results?
20 Feb.	Ask Ian for money he owes me.	Anxious 95% Embarrassed 95% Heart pounding 95% Feeling hot and red 100%	He will shout at me 90% He'll think I'm really mean 90% It will spoil our relationship forever 80% I will have to find another job 80% I won't be able to 70%	There's no evidence he'll react like that. What I know of him shows he's not that kind of person 100% He might be a bit annoyed, but it would pass, and he'd be thinking of something else two minutes later 95%	1. Ask him. Don't apologise or say it doesn't matter. Be polite and pleasant, but firm. Take your time. 2. He gave it to me right away! He said he was sorry, he'd just forgotten.

I'll be stuck at home with no money 70%	Even if he did react like that, everyone would support me. I would if it was someone else. I would think they were entitled to what they were owed 100%		No sign afterwards that he thought anything of it.		
	Maybe I'm entitled too 30%		I learned that if I take the risk, I can get what I want, even if it does make me nervous.		
	Even if I did lose my job, I'm a good enough hairdresser to find another 60%				
	I could be making a mountain out of a molehill here 50%				

Questioning Anxious Predictions Chart

Date/ Time	Situation	Emotions and body sensations Rate 0–100% for intensity.	Anxious predictions Rate belief 0–100%.	Alternative perspectives Use the key questions to find other views of the situation. Rate belief 0–100%.	Outcome 1. What did you do instead of taking your usual precautions? 2. What were the results? 3. What did you learn?

Questioning Anxious Predictions Chart

Date/Time	Situation	Emotions and body sensations Rate 0–100% for intensity.	Anxious predictions Rate belief 0–100%.	Alternative perspectives Use the key questions to find other views of the situation. Rate belief 0–100%.	Outcome 1. What did you do instead of taking your usual precautions? 2. What were the results? 3. What did you learn?

Questioning Anxious Predictions Chart

Date/ Time	Situation	Emotions and body sensations Rate 0–100% for intensity.	Anxious predictions Rate belief 0–100%.	Alternative perspectives Use the key questions to find other views of the situation. Rate belief 0–100%.	Outcome 1. What did you do instead of taking your usual precautions? 2. What were the results? 3. What did you learn?

KEY QUESTIONS

To Help You Find Alternatives to Anxious Predictions

1. What evidence supports what I am predicting?
2. What is the evidence against what I am predicting?
3. What alternative views are there? What evidence is there to support them?
4. What is the worst that can happen?
5. What is the best that can happen?
6. Realistically, what is most likely to happen?
7. If the worst happens, what could be done about it?

Here are some guidelines to help you answer the key questions and fill in your chart.

1 What evidence supports what I am predicting?

- What makes you expect the worst?
- Are there experiences in the past (either recently or earlier in your life) that have led you to expect disaster now?
- Is your main evidence simply your own feelings?
- Or is it just a habit? Do you always automatically expect things to go wrong in this sort of situation? Are you jumping to conclusions, instead of keeping an open mind?

2 What is the evidence against what I am predicting?

- What are the facts of the current situation? Do they support what you think, or do they contradict it?
- In particular, can you find any evidence that does *not* fit your predictions?

- Is there anything you have been ignoring that would suggest that your fears might be exaggerated?
- Are there any resources you could draw on, either in yourself or around you, that you have not been taking into account?
- Have you had any previous experience that suggests things may not go as badly as you fear?

3 What alternative views are there? What evidence supports them?

- How would you view this challenging situation if, for example, you were feeling less anxious and more confident?
- What might another person make of it?
- What would you say to a friend who came to you with the same anxiety – would your predictions be different for them?
- Are you exaggerating the importance of the event?
- How will you see this event after a week? A month? A year? Ten years?
- Will anyone even remember what happened? Will you? If so, will you still feel the same about it?

Write down the alternative perspectives you have found, and then make sure you review the evidence for and against them, just as you reviewed the evidence for and against your original predictions. An alternative that does not fit the facts will not be helpful to you, so make sure that your alternatives are realistic.

4 What is the worst that can happen?

This question is particularly useful in dealing with anxious predictions, because it helps to highlight exaggerations. Look for whatever information you need to obtain a more realistic estimate of the true likelihood of what you fear occurring. Even if it is not impossible, it may be much less likely to happen than you predict.

- Can you visualise the very worst that can happen in vivid detail?
- Does it seem exaggerated or unrealistic?
- Is it likely or even possible?

5 What is the best that can happen?

- Imagine the best possible outcome, to counterbalance your worst. Make it just as positive as your worst is negative.
- Are you less inclined to believe in the best than you were to believe in the worst?
- Why? Could your thinking be biased in some way?

6 Realistically, what is most likely to happen?

- Look at the best and worst possibilities, and see if you can work out, *realistically*, what is actually most likely to happen. (The answer will probably lie somewhere between the best and the worst.)

7 If the worst happens, what could be done about it?

- Just supposing the worst did happen, what personal assets and skills do you have that would help you to deal with it?
- What past experience do you have of successfully dealing with other, similar threats?
- What help, advice and support are available to you from other people?
- What information could you get that would help you to gain a full picture of what is going on and deal more effectively with the situation? Who could you ask? What other sources of information are open to you (e.g. books, social media, people you know)?
- What can you do to change the situation itself? If the situation

that makes you anxious is genuinely unsatisfactory in some way, what changes do you need to make?

Perhaps someone's unreasonable expectations of you need to change, or you need to begin doing more for yourself, or to organise extra help and support. You may well find that such changes are blocked by further negative predictions (e.g. 'But they'll be angry with me') or by self-critical thoughts (e.g. 'But I should be able to cope alone'). If so, make a note of these thoughts and search for alternatives to them. They, too, can be questioned and checked out.

And even if you cannot change the situation itself, it may be possible to make helpful changes in how you react to it. And indeed, that is what you are doing, right now.

How to check out anxious predictions in practice (Core skill 3: Experiments)

Questioning your thoughts may not be enough in itself to convince you that things are better than they seem. You need to act differently, too, to learn how things really are through direct experience. Experimenting with new ways of doing things (for example, being more assertive or accepting challenges you would previously have avoided) enables you to break old habits of thinking and strengthen new ones. These experiments give you an opportunity to find out for yourself whether the alternatives you have found are in line with the facts, and therefore helpful to you, or whether you need to think again. But this will happen only if you take the risk of entering situations you have been avoiding and drop the precautions you have been taking to keep yourself safe.

Decide for yourself where you want to start (when, who with, how?), and the pace you wish to go at. The idea is to find situations that take you out of your comfort zone, but not things that demand too much of you. If you aim too high, anxiety may get in the way of new learning and you may end up disappointed and demoralised.

If you aim too low, however, nothing will change. So, don't try to run before you can walk, but rather go at the pace that best allows you to learn and your confidence to grow.

You can set up experiments deliberately (e.g. planning and carrying out one experiment each day), and you can also use situations that arise without you planning them (e.g. an unexpected phone call or an invitation) to practise acting differently and observing the outcome. Record the results for at least three days, so that you have a chance to experiment in a range of situations. Feel free to continue beyond three days if you feel it would be helpful. Again, the more you practise, the more your confidence will grow.

You can use the **Using Experiments to Check Out Anxious Predictions Chart** on pp. 119–121 to record what you do. (You will see Kate's first experiment in the Outcome column of her 'Questioning Anxious Predictions' chart on p. 106.) You will also find a further blank chart at the back of the book, and you can download them from www.overcoming.co.uk. There are guidelines to help you fill the charts in on pp. 122–125.

Using Experiments to Check Out Anxious Predictions Chart

Date/Time	Situation	Anxious predictions Rate belief 0–100%.	Experiment What will I do instead of taking precautions?	Outcome 1. What have you learned? 2. Were your predictions correct? If not, what perspective would make better sense?

Using Experiments to Check Out Anxious Predictions Chart

Date/Time	Situation	Anxious predictions Rate belief 0–100%.	Experiment What will I do instead of taking precautions?	Outcome 1. What have you learned? 2. Were your predictions correct? If not, what perspective would make better sense?

Using Experiments to Check Out Anxious Predictions Chart

Date/Time	Situation	Anxious predictions Rate belief 0–100%.	Experiment What will I do instead of taking precautions?	Outcome 1. What have you learned? 2. Were your predictions correct? If not, what perspective would make better sense?

Here are some guidelines to help you fill in your chart.

1 State your predictions clearly

It is particularly important to specify your anxious predictions clearly when you come to check them out in action – if your predictions are vague or unclear, you will find it hard to judge whether they are really correct or not. So, as before, write down exactly what you expect to happen, including how you think you will react, and rate each prediction according to how strongly you believe it (from 0 to 100 per cent). For example, if you are predicting that you will feel bad, rate in advance how bad you think you will feel (from 0 to 100 per cent), and in what way. Many people find that, to their surprise, they do indeed feel anxious (for example), but not as much as they expected, especially once they get over the initial hurdle of entering the feared situation. Your rating will give you a chance to find out if this is true for you.

Your predictions may also involve other people's reactions. Perhaps you think that if you behave in a given way, people will lose interest in you, or disapprove of you. If so, how would you know? How would they show that they were indeed losing interest or disapproving? Include comments, gestures, and small signs like changes in facial expression and shifts in direction of gaze. This will tell you exactly what to look for when you go into the situation.

2 What will you do, instead of taking precautions, to ensure that your predictions do not come true?

Use the work you have already done on identifying anxious predictions and precautions to think of all the things you might be tempted to do to protect yourself (no matter how small) and work out in advance what you will do instead. For example:

- If your normal pattern when you talk to someone is to avoid eye contact and say as little as possible about yourself, in case people discover how boring you are, your new pattern might be to look at people and talk as much about yourself as they do about themselves.

- If your normal pattern at work is to have an answer to every question and never admit to ignorance, in case people think you are not up to the job, you could practise sometimes saying 'I don't know' or 'I have no opinion on that'.
- If your normal pattern is to hide your feelings, because to show them at all could lead you to lose control, you might experiment with being a little more open with someone you trust, about something that has upset you, or with showing affection more openly than you normally would.

3 What was the outcome of your experiment?

Always review the results of your experiment afterwards. Ask yourself:

- What did you learn?
- What impact did acting differently have on how you felt?
- How closely did what happened match your original predictions? And how far did it match the alternatives you found?
- What have you discovered about your negative view of yourself – your Bottom Line? Does what happened actually confirm your Bottom Line? Or does the outcome of the experiment suggest that you could afford to think more kindly of yourself?
- And what about your Rules? Does the outcome of this experiment suggest that these have been a good policy to follow all along? Or that it is time for an update?

On the one hand, your experience may show that your anxious predictions were *not* correct, and that the alternatives you found were indeed more realistic and helpful.

On the other hand, your experience may show your anxious predictions to be absolutely correct. If so, do not despair. Provided you remain interested and curious about your experience, you will learn something useful however an experiment turns out. Experiments that 'don't work' often reveal a lot about what is keeping low self-esteem in place. So just ask yourself some more questions:

- How did this come about?
- Was it in fact anything to do with you, or some other element of the situation?
- What other explanations might there be for what went wrong, besides you?
- If you did contribute in some way to what happened, is there any way you could handle the situation differently in future, so as to bring about a different result? For example, are you sure you dropped *all* your precautions? Precautions can be very sneaky; they can creep up on you and catch you unawares. So, watch out for any 'Phew! I just made it!' feelings which will tell you if this has happened.
- If some precautions were still in place, what do you think might have happened if you had dropped them (anxious predictions)? How could you check this out? Exactly what changes do you still need to make to your behaviour?
- How will you ensure that you drop your precautions completely, next time?

When you have carefully thought through what happened, work out what experiments you need to carry out next. Ask yourself:

- How could you apply what you have learned in other situations?
- What further action do you need to take? Each experiment you do does the groundwork for the next, however it turns out. Each discovery is a step on your road to healthy self-esteem.
- Would you find it helpful to repeat the same experiment to build your confidence in the results?
- Or would you prefer to try similar changes in a new and perhaps more challenging situation?

- What does what happened tell you about yourself, other people and how the world works?
- Given what has happened, what predictions would make better sense next time you tackle this type of situation?
- Based on what happened in this particular situation, what general strategies could you adopt to help you deal even more effectively with similar situations in future?

Whatever the outcome of your experiment, congratulate yourself for what you have done. It takes a lot of courage and determination to start facing things you would normally avoid and to do so without your usual precautions. So, whatever the outcome, give yourself a pat on the back. Giving yourself credit for facing challenges is an important part of learning to accept and value yourself, and to discover the freedom to be confidently just who you are.

SUMMARY

1. In situations where your Rules for Living *might* be broken, your Bottom Line is activated and triggers predictions about what could go wrong.
2. Such predictions usually involve: overestimating the chances that something will go wrong; overestimating how bad it would be if it did go wrong; and underestimating your personal resources, and factors outside yourself, which could help to make the situation more manageable.
3. To prevent your predictions from coming true, you take unnecessary precautions which make it impossible to discover if the predictions are correct or not.
4. In order to tackle anxious predictions, you need to learn to spot them as they occur and observe their impact on your emotions and body state, and the unnecessary precautions they lead you to take.

5. The next step is to question your predictions, examining the evidence that supports and contradicts them, and searching for alternative, more realistic perspectives.

6. The final step is to gain direct evidence of how accurate your predictions and your new alternatives are. You can do this by setting up experiments – facing situations that you normally avoid, dropping your unnecessary precautions, and carefully observing the outcome.

SECTION 2:

Questioning Self-Critical Thoughts

This section will help you to understand:

- how self-critical thinking affects you
- why self-critical thinking does more harm than good
- how to become more aware of your self-critical thoughts
- how to question self-critical thoughts
- key questions that can help you find alternatives to self-critical thoughts

How does self-critical thinking affect you?

Tick the responses that most closely match the way you behave when something goes wrong or you make a mistake. Do you usually:

☐ a. call yourself names?

☐ b. tell yourself you should do better?

☐ c. see a single mistake as evidence that you are a stupid/incompetent/inadequate person?

☐ d. ignore the things you got right and concentrate on what you got wrong?

☐ e. blame yourself entirely, ignoring any outside factors that may have caused you to make the mistake?

If you have ticked more than one response, you are behaving in a way that is typical of someone with low self-esteem. People with low self-esteem notice some difficulty, or something wrong about themselves, and on that basis make judgements about themselves as whole people ('stupid', 'incompetent', 'unattractive', 'rotten mother', etc.). These judgements completely ignore the other side of the picture. The end result is a biased point of view, rather than a balanced perspective. The bias expresses itself in self-critical thoughts, which result in painful feelings (sadness, disappointment, anger, guilt), and keep low self-esteem going.

You can get some sense of the emotional impact of self-critical thoughts by carrying out the following experiment. Read the list of words printed below, carefully, allowing each one to sink in.

Imagine they apply to you and notice their impact on your mood. Give each one a score, from 0 (no impact on your mood), through -5 (makes you feel quite bad), to -10 (makes you feel really awful):

Useless _____	Unattractive _____	Incompetent _____
Weak _____	Unlikeable _____	Ugly _____
Pathetic _____	Unwanted _____	Stupid _____
Worthless _____	Inferior _____	Inadequate _____

Some of the words on the list may be familiar to you, from your own self-critical thoughts. If so, put a tick by them. What other words do you use to describe yourself when you are being self-critical? Make a note of them. These are words you will need to watch out for.

In this section you will be able to use the core skills you have already practised in relation to anxious predictions to help you move towards a more balanced and accepting view of yourself. You will be learning to become aware of self-critical thinking as it happens, and to observe carefully its impact on your feelings and how you behave in day-to-day situations.

This is the part of the vicious circle we shall be working on:

How self-criticism keeps low self-esteem going

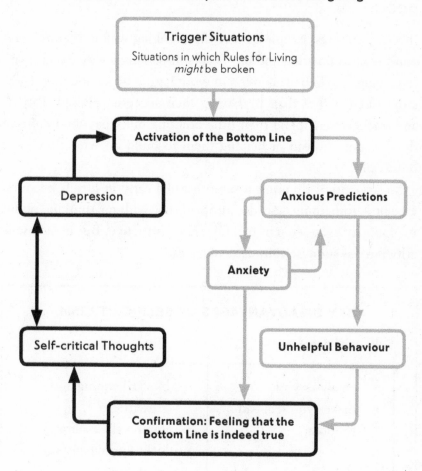

You will learn how to question self-critical thoughts, just as you learned to question your anxious predictions, and to search for kinder and fairer alternatives. Then in Section 3 we shall turn to the other side of the equation: learning to become more aware of positive aspects of yourself, to give more weight to your strengths, assets, qualities and talents, and to treat yourself with the same consideration you would give another person you cared about.

Why self-critical thinking does more harm than good

In many cultures, people believe that thinking well of themselves is equivalent to boasting and big-headedness. This is why children are often taught to behave better and work harder by having their faults emphasised, rather than by having their successes praised. Parents and teachers may spend their time pointing out what children have done wrong, instead of helping them to build on what they have done right.

So self-critical thinking is often learned early in life. It becomes a habit – something you do automatically without thinking about it. You may even see it as helpful and constructive. But in fact, self-criticism has some serious disadvantages.

KEY DISADVANTAGES OF SELF-CRITICISM

Self-criticism:

• paralyses you • makes you feel bad • is unfair	• blocks learning and growth • ignores the realities • kicks you when you are down

---

Self-criticism paralyses you and makes you feel bad

Imagine a person you know who is quite self-confident. Imagine following them around, pointing out every little mistake they make, calling them names, telling them what they have done is all very well but could have been done better/faster/more effectively. As the days and weeks went by, what effect would you expect this constant drip, drip, drip of criticism to have?

How would they feel?

_____

_____

_____

_____

How would it affect their confidence?

_____

_____

_____

_____

_____

How would it influence their ability to make decisions?

_____

_____

_____

_____

_____

Would it make life easier for them, or more difficult?

_____

_____

_____

_____

_____

Would you even consider doing this to a friend of yours?

_____

_____

_____

_____

If not, why not?

_____

_____

_____

_____

_____

_____

_____

If you have the habit of self-critical thinking, then this is probably what you are doing to yourself, perhaps without even being particularly aware of it. Self-critical thoughts are like a parrot on your shoulder, constantly squawking disapproval in your ear. Consider how this may be discouraging and demoralising you and paralysing your efforts to change and grow.

Self-criticism is unfair

Being self-critical means that you react to mistakes, failures or errors of judgement – even very small ones – as if they told the whole story about you. When you notice a single fault or weakness, you use it as a reason to tell yourself you are bad, pathetic or stupid *as a person*.

Do you think this is fair? _____

Would you think it was fair to treat another person in the same way?

_____

When you condemn yourself as a person on the basis of an error or something you regret, you are drawing a general conclusion about yourself on the basis of biased evidence, taking only negative aspects of yourself into account. Be realistic: give yourself credit for your assets and strengths as well as acknowledging that, like the rest of the human race, you have weaknesses and flaws.

Self-critical thinking blocks learning and growth

Self-criticism undermines your confidence and makes you feel discouraged, demoralised and bad about yourself.

How much will this help you to overcome your problems, and alter those aspects of yourself that you genuinely want to change?

_____

_____

_____

_____

Does self-criticism give you any clues as to how to do better next time?

_____

_____

_____

_____

Do you think people learn more when their successes are praised or when they are punished for their failures?

_____

_____

_____

_____

If you pay attention only to what you do wrong, you lose the opportunity to learn from and repeat what you do right. Similarly, if you write yourself off every time you make an error, you lose the opportunity to learn from your mistakes and to work constructively on aspects of yourself that you wish to change.

Self-critical thinking ignores the realities

When things go wrong, in addition to criticising yourself for what you did, you probably tell yourself you *should* have acted differently. With hindsight, it is often easy to see how you could have handled things better. But how did things appear to you *at the time*?

Think of a specific time when this was the case. What was happening?

_____

_____

_____

_____

_____

How were you feeling?

_____

_____

_____

_____

_____

Were you thinking clearly?

_____

_____

_____

_____

_____

Did you have all the information you needed to deal with the situation in the best possible way?

_____

_____

_____

_____

_____

Taking all these circumstances into account, it's probably completely understandable that you acted as you did, even if it turned out not to be in your best interests. This does not mean letting yourself off the hook if you genuinely did do something you regret. But you can learn from experiences by looking back at them. Then, if a similar situation arises again, you will have a different perspective on how to deal with it. Punishing yourself by brooding on past mistakes will only make you feel bad. It will not help you to think more clearly and do better next time.

Self-critical thinking kicks you when you are down

People with low self-esteem sometimes criticise themselves for the problems they are experiencing (e.g. anxiety, depression, lack of assertiveness). They may even criticise themselves for not being more self-confident. This lack of compassion ignores the fact that we all have difficulties of one kind or another, and that they are normally an understandable result of our experiences in life. It just makes you feel even more undermined and demoralised.

If another person had experienced the difficulties you have encountered in your life, what sort of problems might they have?

_____

_____

_____

_____

_____

Is it possible that your difficulties (including how you think about yourself) are a natural reaction to distressing events?

_____

_____

_____

_____

_____

If someone you cared about had similar difficulties, developed under the same circumstances, what advice would you give to him or her?

_____

_____

_____

_____

_____

Very likely, anyone who had experienced what you have experienced would see themselves as you do. With the help of this handbook, and other resources if necessary, you will be able to find ways to manage self-critical thinking and its consequences more successfully. What is certain is that criticising yourself for having difficulties will not help you to resolve them.

Questioning self-critical thoughts

It is clear from this that self-critical thinking can be damaging. How then to tackle it?

The skills involved are the same core skills you practised when you were finding out how to question and test anxious predictions in the previous section. They are:

- **1. Awareness**: Learning to catch self-critical thoughts as they happen
- **2. Re-thinking:** Questioning self-critical thoughts and looking for more realistic and helpful alternatives
- **3. Experiments**: Practising viewing yourself more compassionately and behaving accordingly

1 Awareness: How to become more familiar with your self-critical thoughts

The first step is to notice when you put yourself down, and to observe what impact it has on how you feel and behave. Your emotions can be a signal that self-critical thinking is going on. For this reason, it is helpful to learn to recognise them when they occur.

Think of a time when you did something you regretted: When and where did the incident happen?

_____

_____

_____

_____

_____

Who was there?

_____

_____

_____

_____

_____

What happened?

_____

_____

_____

_____

What did you say to yourself afterwards?

_____

_____

_____

_____

Tick the feelings you experienced:

☐ Guilty	☐ Ashamed
☐ Sad	☐ Embarrassed
☐ Disappointed in yourself	☐ Angry with yourself
☐ Frustrated	☐ Depressed
☐ Hopeless	☐ Despairing

Filling in a **Spotting Self-Critical Thoughts Chart** (see pp. 145–152) will help you to notice what is running through your mind when you feel bad about yourself, and to understand more clearly how these thoughts keep the vicious circle of low self-esteem going. As before, see if you can bring a spirit of interest and curiosity to your investigations. You may well find that the same thoughts (or very similar ones) occur again and again. There is another blank chart at the back of the book, which you can photocopy if you wish, and it can also be downloaded from www.overcoming.co.uk.

Let's take Mike, from Part One of this handbook, as an example of how to keep this kind of record. You may remember that Mike accidentally knocked down and killed a woman who stepped off the pavement in front of him. At one point, after several months of being troubled by what happened, Mike had a few days of feeling considerably better. The accident seemed to be playing on his mind rather less, and he had been feeling more relaxed, more on top of things and more like his normal self.

Then, one day, his daughter was very late home from school. Mike was terrified. He was certain something terrible had happened to her. In fact, he had forgotten that she was going to a friend's house. When she came in, he went ballistic. Afterwards, he felt thoroughly ashamed of himself. What a way to behave! 'This proves it,' he thought. 'I am really losing it. I'm a total mess.' He felt more and more upset. 'Pull yourself together,' he said to himself. 'This is pathetic. Get a grip.' The episode confirmed his worst suspicions about himself: he *was* a nervous wreck, there was no doubt about it. And there seemed little chance of change. Mike was just about ready to give up.

You will find Mike's completed chart over the page.

Spotting Self-Critical Thoughts Chart: Mike

Date/Time	Situation What were you doing when you began to feel bad about yourself?	Emotions and body sensations (e.g. sad, angry, guilty, tense). Rate each 0–100 for intensity.	Self-critical thoughts What exactly was going through your mind when you began to feel bad about yourself (e.g. thoughts in words, images, meanings)? Rate belief in each one 0–100%.	Unhelpful behaviour What did you do as a consequence of your self-critical thoughts?
5 March	Got in a rage with Kelly when she came home late. Had completely forgotten she was going to Jan's house.	Guilty 80 Fed up with myself 100 Hopeless 95	This proves it – I'm really losing it 100% I'm a total mess 95% I should pull myself together 100% This is pathetic 100% What's the matter with me? I just don't think I'll ever get back to how I was 95%	Stomped out of the house and went to the pub. Came back late and shut myself in the basement alone to watch TV. Didn't talk to anyone.

The Spotting Self-Critical Thoughts Chart

The best way to tune in to self-critical thoughts is to make a note of them as soon as they occur. This is the first step to questioning them and searching for more helpful and realistic alternatives, just as you did with anxious predictions. Over the course of a few days, completing the chart will help you to recognise the changes in your feelings that signal the presence of self-critical thoughts.

Keep your record for about a week, filling in one chart every day. By then, you should have a pretty good idea of the kind of situations that spark self-critical thinking, and its impact on your emotions and what you do. Here are some guidelines to help you fill in the charts:

Date and time

- When did you feel bad about yourself?

Over time, you can use this information to pick up repeating patterns, as you did with your anxious predictions.

The situation

- What was happening at the moment you began to feel bad about yourself?
- Where were you?
- Who were you with?
- What were you doing?

Briefly describe what was going on (e.g. 'asked a girl out – she turned me down' or 'boss asked me to rewrite a report'). Perhaps you weren't doing anything in particular (e.g. washing up or watching television), and your self-critical thinking was triggered by something in your own mind. In this case, write down the general topic you were focusing on (e.g. 'thinking about my ex-husband taking the children for the weekend' or 'remembering being bullied at school'). Your exact thoughts, word for word, belong in the 'Self-critical thoughts' column.

Emotions and body sensations

- Did you feel one main emotion (e.g. sadness)?
- Or did you experience a mixture of emotions (e.g. not only sadness, but also guilt and anger)?
- Did you also experience changes in your body state (e.g. a sinking feeling or a churning stomach)?

Rate each emotion and body sensation between 0 and 100, according to how strong it was. (A rating of 5 would mean just a very faint emotional reaction or physical change; a rating of 50 would mean a moderate level of distress; and a rating of 100 would mean the emotion or sensation was as strong as it could possibly be.)

Self-critical thoughts

- What was running through your mind when you began to feel bad about yourself?
- Did you hear a voice in your mind, calling you names or telling you that you should have done better?
- Or did your thoughts take the form of images in your mind's eye?
- If you cannot identify any particular thoughts or images, ask: what does this situation mean to you? What does it tell you about yourself? What does it imply about what others think of you? What does it say about your future?

Rate each self-critical thought, image or meaning between 0 per cent and 100 per cent, according to how far you believed it when it occurred. (A rating of 100 per cent would mean you believed it completely, with no shadow of doubt; 50 per cent would mean you were in two minds; 5 per cent would mean you only believed it slightly.)

Unhelpful behaviour

What impact did your self-critical thoughts have on your behaviour? For example:
- Did you apologise for yourself?
- Did you withdraw into your shell?
- Did you avoid asking for something you needed?
- Did you allow yourself to be treated like a doormat or ignored?
- Did you avoid an opportunity that you might otherwise have taken?

On pp. 153–154 you will find the most frequently asked questions about the **Spotting Self-Critical Thoughts Chart**.

Spotting Self-Critical Thoughts Chart

Date/Time	Situation What were you doing when you began to feel bad about yourself?	Emotions and body sensations (e.g. sad, angry, guilty, tense). Rate each 0–100 for intensity.	Self-critical thoughts What exactly was going through your mind when you began to feel bad about yourself (e.g. thoughts in words, images, meanings)? Rate belief in each one 0–100%.	Unhelpful behaviour What did you do as a consequence of your self-critical thoughts?

Spotting Self-Critical Thoughts Chart

Date/Time	Situation What were you doing when you began to feel bad about yourself?	Emotions and body sensations (e.g. sad, angry, guilty, tense). Rate each 0–100 for intensity.	Self-critical thoughts What exactly was going through your mind when you began to feel bad about yourself (e.g. thoughts in words, images, meaning)? Rate belief in each one 0–100%.	Unhelpful behaviour What did you do as a consequence of your self-critical thoughts?

Spotting Self-Critical Thoughts Chart

Date/Time	Situation What were you doing when you began to feel bad about yourself?	Emotions and body sensations (e.g. sad, angry, guilty, tense). Rate each 0–100 for intensity.	Self-critical thoughts What exactly was going through your mind when you began to feel bad about yourself (e.g. thoughts in words, images, meanings)? Rate belief in each one 0–100%.	Unhelpful behaviour What did you do as a consequence of your self-critical thoughts?

Spotting Self-Critical Thoughts Chart

Date/Time	Situation What were you doing when you began to feel bad about yourself?	Emotions and body sensations (e.g. sad, angry, guilty, tense). Rate each 0–100 for intensity.	Self-critical thoughts What exactly was going through your mind when you began to feel bad about yourself (e.g. thoughts in words, images, meanings)? Rate belief in each one 0–100%.	Unhelpful behaviour What did you do as a consequence of your self-critical thoughts?

Spotting Self-Critical Thoughts Chart

Date/Time	Situation What were you doing when you began to feel bad about yourself?	Emotions and body sensations (e.g. sad, angry, guilty, tense). Rate each 0–100 for intensity.	Self-critical thoughts What exactly was going through your mind when you began to feel bad about yourself (e.g. thoughts in words, images, meanings)? Rate belief in each one 0–100%.	Unhelpful behaviour What did you do as a consequence of your self-critical thoughts?

Spotting Self-Critical Thoughts Chart

| Date/Time | Situation

What were you doing when you began to feel bad about yourself? | Emotions and body sensations

(e.g. sad, angry, guilty, tense).

Rate each 0–100 for intensity. | Self-critical thoughts

What exactly was going through your mind when you began to feel bad about yourself

(e.g. thoughts in words, images, meanings)? Rate belief in each one 0–100%. | Unhelpful behaviour

What did you do as a consequence of your self-critical thoughts? |
|---|---|---|---|---|
| | | | | |
| | | | | |

Spotting Self-Critical Thoughts Chart

Date/Time	Situation What were you doing when you began to feel bad about yourself?	Emotions and body sensations (e.g. sad, angry, guilty, tense). Rate each 0–100 for intensity.	Self-critical thoughts What exactly was going through your mind when you began to feel bad about yourself (e.g. thoughts in words, images, meanings)? Rate belief in each one 0–100%.	Unhelpful behaviour What did you do as a consequence of your self-critical thoughts?

Spotting Self-Critical Thoughts Chart

Date/Time	Situation What were you doing when you began to feel bad about yourself?	Emotions and body sensations (e.g. sad, angry, guilty, tense). Rate each 0–100 for intensity.	Self-critical thoughts What exactly was going through your mind when you began to feel bad about yourself (e.g. thoughts in words, images, meanings)? Rate belief in each one 0–100%.	Unhelpful behaviour What did you do as a consequence of your self-critical thoughts?

Frequently asked questions about the Spotting the Self-Critical Thoughts Chart

Here are some of the questions people often ask about filling in the **Spotting Self-Critical Thoughts Chart**.

Why bother to write things down?

Having a record in black and white can help you to stay in touch with what actually happens. You will have something concrete to reflect on, and there is less chance of you forgetting the detail of incidents. You can notice repeating patterns, consider how your thoughts affect your behaviour in different situations, and become aware of the exact words you use to yourself when you are being self-critical.

Equally, people often find that, if you write your thoughts down, it can take them out of your head (so to speak), and allow you to stand back from them, take a good look at them and gain a different perspective. This will help you to move towards the point where you can begin to say, 'Aha, there's another one of those!' and to see them as something you do, rather than a true reflection of yourself.

How many thoughts do I need to record?

The key thing is to gain a clear understanding of your personal patterns of self-criticism and their impact on your life, the things that come up again and again for you. You could start by noting one or two self-critical thoughts each day. When noticing them and observing their impact has become fairly automatic, you will be ready to move on to finding alternatives to your self-critical thoughts. This could take up to a week – but you may find you get the hang of it more quickly than that, or on the other hand that you may need a bit more time.

When should I make the record?

As with anxious predictions, the ideal is to record your self-critical thoughts as soon as they occur. This means keeping your record with you. The reason for this is that, although self-critical thoughts can have a very powerful effect when they actually occur, it may be hard afterwards to remember exactly what ran through your mind, especially if you were very distressed at the time.

Of course, the ideal is not always possible. If you cannot record what happened at the time, make sure that at least you make a careful mental note of what upset you, or jot down a reminder on your phone or a notepad, or on any handy piece of paper. Then set aside time later to make a proper, detailed written record. Run through an 'action replay' in your mind – remember as vividly as you can where you were and what you were doing, the moment when you started to feel bad about yourself, what was running through your mind at that moment, and what you did in response to your thoughts.

Won't focusing on my self-critical thoughts just upset me?

It is natural to want to avoid focusing on upsetting ideas. You may feel understandably reluctant to record these damning judgements of yourself in black and white. But if you want to tackle your self-critical thoughts effectively, you first need to look them in the face. So, beware of excuses ('I'll do it later', 'It doesn't do to dwell on things'). Making excuses will deprive you of the chance to develop a more kindly perspective on yourself. And ignoring the thoughts will not make them go away.

2 Re-thinking: How to question your self-critical thoughts and find fairer, more helpful alternatives

Developing awareness of your self-critical thoughts is the first step towards questioning them. The aim is to stop taking your self-critical thoughts as if they were statements of the truth about yourself, and to begin to find alternative perspectives that will provide you with a more balanced view.

You can use the **Questioning Self-Critical Thoughts Chart** to help you do this. You will find one of Mike's completed charts on p. 156 as an illustration.

You will see that the first four columns of this sheet are identical to **Spotting Self-Critical Thoughts** (date/time; situation; emotions/body sensations; self-critical thoughts). However, the new chart does not stop there. Mike has also been asked to record 'alternative perspectives' (re-thinking) and 'outcome' (just as you did when you questioned your anxious predictions). Notice too that 'Outcome' includes an action question (experiments).

On pp. 174–77 there are some more guidelines and frequently asked questions to help you fill in these extra columns on your own **Questioning Self-Critical Thoughts Charts** on pp. 158–71. There is another blank chart at the back of the handbook, which you can photocopy if you wish, and of course it can be downloaded from www.overcoming.co.uk.

Alternative perspectives

On p. 172 you will find a list of Key Questions designed to help you to explore alternative perspectives. Rate each alternative according to how far you believe it, just as you rated the original self-critical thoughts (100 per cent if you believe it completely, 0 per cent if you do not believe it at all, and so on). You do not have to believe all your answers 100 per cent. They should, however, be convincing enough to make at least some difference to how you feel. Each question is discussed in more detail later, on pp. 178–83.

Questioning Self-Critical Thoughts Chart: Mike

Date/Time	Situation	Emotions and body sensations Rate each 0–100 for intensity.	Self-critical thoughts Rate belief in each 0–100%.	Alternative perspectives Use the key questions to find other perspectives on yourself. Rate belief in each one 0–100%.	Outcome 1. Now that you have found alternatives to your self-critical thoughts, how do you feel (0–100)? 2. How far do you now believe the self-critical thoughts (0–100%)? 3. What can you do (action plan, experiments)?
8 March	Had a row with Kelly again. She wanted to go out on a friend's motorbike.	Guilty 80 Angry with myself 100 Hopeless 90	Here I go again losing my temper over nothing. I am a wreck 100% I've got to get a grip on myself or I'll ruin everything 100%	It's true that I was angrier than the situation warranted. But it's because I get frightened for her. Bikes are quite dangerous and I'm afraid of losing her. So, it wasn't really about nothing. 100%	1. Guilty 40 Angry with self 30 Hopeless 40 2. 30% 20% 50%

<table>
</table>

3. Tell Kelly I'm sorry about shouting at her and explain why

Talk to Viv (my wife) and tell her how I feel instead of shutting her out.

Get help?

I do need to do something about all this, it's true. I have changed a lot. But then, I went through something really bad, so maybe it's not surprising I'm not my usual self. 90%

Rows are not good for any of us. But in fact, we usually get over it. She's a good girl, even if a bit of a cranky teenager at the moment. We have some good times together. 95%

I don't know how to answer that. It's been going on a while. I don't like doing it, but maybe it's time to get help. 50%

There's no end to this 90%

Questioning Self-Critical Thoughts Chart

Date/ Time	Situation	Emotions and body sensations Rate each 0–100 for intensity.	Self-critical thoughts Rate belief in each 0–100%.	Alternative perspectives Use the key questions to find other perspectives on yourself. Rate belief in each one 0–100%.	Outcome 1. Now that you have found alternatives to your self-critical thoughts, how do you feel (0–100)? 2. How far do you now believe the self-critical thoughts (0–100%)? 3. What can you do (action plan, experiments)?

Questioning Self-Critical Thoughts Chart

Date/Time	Situation	Emotions and body sensations Rate each 0–100 for intensity.	Self-critical thoughts Rate belief in each 0–100%.	Alternative perspectives Use the key questions to find other perspectives on yourself. Rate belief in each one 0–100%.	Outcome 1. Now that you have found alternatives to your self-critical thoughts, how do you feel (0–100)? 2. How far do you now believe the self-critical thoughts (0–100%)? 3. What can you do (action plan, experiments)?

Questioning Self-Critical Thoughts Chart

Date/ Time	Situation	Emotions and body sensations Rate each 0–100 for intensity.	Self-critical thoughts Rate belief in each 0–100%.	Alternative perspectives Use the key questions to find other perspectives on yourself. Rate belief in each one 0–100%.	Outcome 1. Now that you have found alternatives to your self-critical thoughts, how do you feel (0–100)? 2. How far do you now believe the self-critical thoughts (0–100%)? 3. What can you do (action plan, experiments)?

Questioning Self-Critical Thoughts Chart

Date/ Time	Situation	Emotions and body sensations Rate each 0–100 for intensity.	Self-critical thoughts Rate belief in each 0–100%.	Alternative perspectives Use the key questions to find other perspectives on yourself. Rate belief in each one 0–100%.	Outcome 1. Now that you have found alternatives to your self-critical thoughts, how do you feel (0–100)? 2. How far do you now believe the self-critical thoughts (0–100%)? 3. What can you do (action plan, experiments)?

Questioning Self-Critical Thoughts Chart

Date/ Time	Situation	Emotions and body sensations Rate each 0–100 for intensity.	Self-critical thoughts Rate belief in each 0–100%.	Alternative perspectives Use the key questions to find other perspectives on yourself. Rate belief in each one 0–100%.	Outcome 1. Now that you have found alternatives to your self-critical thoughts, how do you feel (0–100)? 2. How far do you now believe the self-critical thoughts (0–100%)? 3. What can you do (action plan, experiments)?

Questioning Self-Critical Thoughts Chart

Date/ Time	Situation	Emotions and body sensations Rate each 0–100 for intensity.	Self-critical thoughts Rate belief in each 0–100%.	Alternative perspectives Use the key questions to find other perspectives on yourself. Rate belief in each one 0–100%.	Outcome 1. Now that you have found alternatives to your self-critical thoughts, how do you feel (0–100)? 2. How far do you now believe the self-critical thoughts (0–100%)? 3. What can you do (action plan, experiments)?

Questioning Self-Critical Thoughts Chart

Date/ Time	Situation	Emotions and body sensations Rate each 0–100 for intensity.	Self-critical thoughts Rate belief in each 0–100%.	Alternative perspectives Use the key questions to find other perspectives on yourself. Rate belief in each one 0–100%.	Outcome 1. Now that you have found alternatives to your self-critical thoughts, how do you feel (0–100)? 2. How far do you now believe the self-critical thoughts (0–100%)? 3. What can you do (action plan, experiments)?

KEY QUESTIONS

To Help You Find Alternatives to Self-Critical Thoughts

1. **What is the evidence?**
   - Am I confusing a thought with a fact?
   - What is the evidence in favour of my self-critical thoughts?
   - What is the evidence against my self-critical thoughts?

2. **What alternative perspectives are there?**
   - Am I assuming my perspective is the only one possible?
   - What evidence do I have to support alternative perspectives?

3. **What is the effect of thinking the way I do about myself?**
   - Are these self-critical thoughts helpful to me, or are they getting in my way?
   - What perspective might be more helpful to me?

4. **What are the biases in my thinking about myself?**
   - Am I jumping to conclusions?
   - Am I using a double standard?
   - Am I thinking in all-or-nothing terms?
   - Am I condemning myself as a total person on the basis of a single event?
   - Am I concentrating on my weaknesses and forgetting my strengths?
   - Am I blaming myself for things which are not really my fault?
   - Am I expecting myself to be perfect?

5. **What can I do?**
   - How can I put a new, kinder perspective into practice?
   - Is there anything I need to do to change the situation? Even if not, what can I do to change my own thinking about it in future?
   - How can I experiment with acting in a less self-defeating way?

Outcome

Go back to your original emotions and body sensations. How strong are they now? Rate each one out of 100 per cent for intensity. Then go back to your original self-critical thoughts. Having found alternatives to them, how far do you now believe them? Rate each 1 to 100 per cent according to how far you believe it *now*.

If your answers have been effective, you should find that your belief in the self-critical thoughts, together with the painful emotions that go with them, has lessened to some extent.

Action

The question here is: What can I do now to put my new perspective into practice in everyday life, and treat myself more compassionately? This is the third skill you learned when you were checking out your anxious predictions through direct experience, that is, experiments. Remember: experience is the best teacher and you will find your alternatives most convincing if you have acted on them and discovered for yourself how they change your feelings and the possibilities open to you.

Frequently asked questions about the Questioning Self-Critical Thoughts Chart

Before we explore each of the key questions on the list on p. 172 in detail, let us first consider how to go about the process of questioning your self-critical thoughts effectively. Here are some of the issues people often raise about the **Questioning Self-Critical Thoughts Chart**.

How long will it take to find good alternatives to my self-critical thoughts?

The habit of self-criticism takes time to break. Changing your thinking is rather like taking up a new form of exercise. You are being asked to develop mental muscles you do not normally use. They will feel awkward and uncomfortable at first. But, with regular practice, they will become strong, flexible and able to do what you require of them. The objective at this stage is to reach the point where you automatically notice, question and dismiss self-critical thoughts. Regular daily practice (one or two written examples a day) is the best way to achieve this. You may find it takes you about a week to get the hang of answering self-critical thoughts – or it may take longer. Don't rush it – give yourself time to practise, learn from your mistakes, and develop your re-thinking skill. Learning to be fair and kind to yourself is central to cultivating healthy self-esteem.

Later, you will be able to find answers to self-critical thoughts in your head without needing to record anything. Eventually, you may find that most of the time you do not even need to answer thoughts in your head – they no longer occur very much. And even when they do pop up, you no longer believe them strongly. Even so, you may still find the record sheet helpful when dealing with particularly tough thoughts, or at times when you are pressured or unhappy for some reason. In short, regular daily recordings need only go on until you achieve the objective of being able to deal with self-critical thoughts without a written prompt.

How can I expect to think differently when I'm feeling really upset?

Self-critical thoughts reflect the voice of your low self-esteem. This means that they can be loud, compelling and charged with emotion. It does not follow that they are true, and now you are learning to distance yourself from them, to stop buying into them and taking them seriously.

If something happens that upsets you deeply, it will probably be very difficult to find alternatives to your self-critical thoughts. Instead of grasping that this is a common, natural difficulty, you may fall into the trap of seeing it as yet another reason to criticise yourself. The most helpful thing to do is simply to make a note of what happened to upset you, and your feelings and thoughts, but then to leave the search for alternatives until you are feeling calmer. You will be in a better position to see things clearly after you have weathered the storm.

Beware the rumination trap

Sometimes self-critical thinking consists of a simple judgement: 'You idiot', 'Why do I never get anything right?' But unless you spot it, it can easily shade into rumination, brooding – going over and over the same thing, round and round, again and again, like a cow chewing the cud. Streams of 'whys', 'if onlys', unfair self-judgements, harping on endlessly about the gap between who you are and who you want to be or think you should be ('It/I should be different' thinking). This can feel like a helpful problem-solving strategy: maybe if I go round the block one more time, I will find the answer. But in fact, it has just the opposite effect. Rumination just leads to more rumination and makes you miserable, especially if your mood is already low.

So, if you notice your mind is following the same old track over and over again, it's time to make a choice. You can choose to continue ruminating, in the hopes that in the end you'll get somewhere. Or you could decide to experiment with deliberately placing your attention elsewhere (for example, engaging in an absorbing activity, or deliberately thinking about something else). You cannot stop thoughts from coming into your mind, but you can influence what happens next. See if you can learn to let your ruminations be like a radio in the background – you can still tune in to the programme if you wish, but most of the time you have better things to do.

How good does the record have to be?

Many people with low self-esteem are perfectionists. However, it is important to bear in mind the purpose of the record: increasing self-awareness and increasing flexibility in your thinking. Taking a perfectionist approach won't help you to achieve this – it will only create pressure to perform, and stifle creativity. You do not have to find the one *right* answer, or the answer you think you *should* put. The 'right' answer is the answer that makes sense to you and changes your feelings for the better. No answer, however sensible it may seem, will work for everyone. You need to find the answers that work best for *you*.

What if my alternatives don't work?

Sometimes people find that the answers they come up with make little difference to how they feel and act. If this is the case for you, perhaps you are disqualifying the answer in some way – maybe telling yourself that it applies to other people, but not to you? If you have 'yes, buts' like this, write them down in the 'Self-critical thoughts' column and question them. Do not expect your belief in your old thoughts and painful feelings to shrink to zero right away, especially if they reflect beliefs about yourself which have been in place for many years. Self-critical thinking can be like a pair of old shoes – not very pleasant, but familiar and moulded to your shape. New perspectives, in contrast, are like new shoes – unfamiliar and stiff. You will need time to practise 'walking in them' until they start to feel comfortable. And you will need to experiment repeatedly with acting differently towards yourself, so that you learn on a gut level that compassion and self-acceptance work better for you than self-criticism.

What if I'm no good at this?

Don't allow yourself to get caught in the trap of self-criticism while you are recording your self-critical thoughts. Changing how you think about yourself is no easy task. So, beware of being hard on yourself when you find the going tough. If you had a friend who was trying to tackle something difficult, would it be more helpful to praise or to criticise them? You may catch yourself thinking 'I must be really stupid to think this way' or 'I'm not doing enough of this' or 'I will never get the hang of this'. If you do spot thoughts like these – write them down and answer them. And see if as you do this you can learn to give yourself the respect and encouragement you would give to a good friend who was attempting a difficult task.

Key questions to help you find helpful alternatives to self-critical thoughts

The questions listed on p. 172 and detailed below are designed to help you explore fresh perspectives and recognise how your self-critical thoughts are not only biased and one-sided, but also unhelpful and unkind. At first, you may find it useful to use the whole list. Then, as you go along, you will notice which questions seem particularly helpful in tackling your own personal style of self-critical thinking. You could write down these especially helpful questions on a card small enough to carry in your wallet or purse, or perhaps store them on your mobile phone or tablet, and use them to free up your thinking when self-critical thoughts strike. With practice, useful questions will become part of your mental furniture. At that point, you will no longer need a written prompt.

1 What is the evidence?

Am I confusing a thought with a fact?

Just because you believe something to be true, it does not follow that it is. I could believe that I am a giraffe. But would that make me one? Your self-critical thoughts may be opinions based on unfortunate experiences you have had, not a reflection of your true self.

What is the evidence in favour of my self-critical thoughts?

What are you going on, when you judge yourself critically? What actual evidence do you have to support what you think of yourself? What facts or observations (rather than ideas or opinions) back up your self-critical thoughts?

What is the evidence against my self-critical thoughts?

Can you think of anything that suggests that your poor opinion of yourself is not completely true? Or indeed contradicts it? Finding counter-evidence may not be easy, because you will tend to screen it out or discount it. This does not mean it does not exist. It may be helpful to discuss this with a trusted friend or supporter – they may have a clearer, fairer view of you than you have of yourself.

2 What alternative perspectives are there?

Am I assuming that my perspective on myself is the only one possible?

Any situation can be viewed from many different angles. How would you see this particular situation on a day when you were feeling more confident and on top of things? How do you think you will view it in ten years' time? What would you say if a friend of yours came to you with this problem? And what would your friend say if they knew what you were thinking? Would they agree? If your loss of confidence has been relatively recent, how would you have viewed the situation before the difficulty began?

Remember to check out alternative perspectives against available evidence. An alternative with no basis in reality will not be helpful to you.

3 What is the effect of thinking the way I do about myself?

Are these self-critical thoughts helpful to me, or are they getting in my way?

What are your goals or objectives in this specific situation? How do you *want* things to turn out? Right now, do the disadvantages of self-critical thinking outweigh its advantages? Is it the best way to get what you want out of the situation, or would a more balanced, kindly, encouraging perspective be more helpful? Are your self-critical thoughts helping you to handle things constructively, or are they encouraging self-defeating behaviour?

4 What are the biases in my thinking about myself?

Am I jumping to conclusions?

This means deciding how things are, without proper evidence to support your point of view – for example, concluding that the fact that someone didn't call you means that you must have done something to offend them, when actually you have no idea why they haven't called. People with low self-esteem typically jump to whatever conclusion reflects badly on themselves. Is this a habit of yours? If so, remember to review the evidence, the facts. When you look at the bigger picture, you may discover that your critical conclusion about yourself is incorrect.

Am I using a double standard?

People with low self-esteem are often much harder on themselves than they would be on anyone else. To find out if you are using a double standard, ask yourself what your reaction would be if someone you cared about came to you with a problem. Would you tell them that they were weak or stupid or pathetic, or that they should know better? Or would you be encouraging and sympathetic and try to help them to get the problem into perspective and look for constructive ways of dealing with it? Try taking a step back from your usual critical and disapproving stance and experiment with being kind, sympathetic and encouraging to yourself, just as you would to another person. You may well find that in fact treating yourself more kindly makes you feel better and helps you to think clearly and act constructively.

Am I thinking in all-or-nothing terms?

All-or-nothing, 'either/or' thinking oversimplifies things. In fact, nearly everything is relative. So, for example, people are not usually all good or all bad, but a mixture of the two. Events are not usually complete disasters or total successes, but somewhere in the middle. Are you thinking about yourself in all-or-nothing terms? The words you use may be a clue here. Watch out for extreme words (always/never, everyone/no one, everything/nothing). They may reflect all-or-nothing thinking. In fact, things are probably less clear-cut than that. So, look for the shades of grey.

Am I condemning myself as a total person on the basis of a single event?

People with low self-esteem commonly make global judgements about themselves on the basis of one thing they said or did, or one problem they have. Are you making this kind of blanket judgement about yourself? One person dislikes you, and it must mean there is something wrong with you? One mistake, and you are a failure?

Judging yourself as a total person on the basis of any single thing does not make sense. If you did one thing really well, would that make you totally wonderful as a person? You probably wouldn't even dream of thinking so. But when it comes to your weaknesses and mistakes, you may be only too ready to write yourself off.

You need to look at the bigger picture. And remember that when you are feeling down, you will be homing in on anything that fits with your poor opinion of yourself and screening out anything that does not fit. This biases your judgement even more. So, hold back from making global judgements, unless you are sure that you are taking all the evidence into account.

Am I concentrating on my weaknesses and forgetting my strengths?

People with low self-esteem commonly overlook problems they have successfully handled in the past and forget their good qualities and the personal resources that could help them to overcome current difficulties. Do you tend to focus on things that go wrong, and ignore anything you have enjoyed or achieved?

Of course, there are things you are not very good at, things you have done that you regret, and things about yourself that you would prefer to change. This is true for every normal, imperfect human being. But what about the other side of the equation? What are the things you *are* good at? What do other people appreciate about you? What do you like about yourself? How have you coped with difficulties and stresses in your life? What are your strengths, qualities and resources? (We shall return to this in detail in Section 3.)

Am I blaming myself for things which are not really my fault?

When things go wrong, do you consider all the possible reasons why this might be so, or do you immediately assume that it must be due to some failing in yourself? If a friend stands you up, for example, do you automatically assume that you must have done something to annoy them?

There are all kinds of reasons why things do not work out. Sometimes, of course, it will indeed be a result of something you did. But often, other factors are involved. For example, your friend might have forgotten, or been exceptionally busy, or have misunderstood your arrangements. If you automatically assume responsibility when things go wrong, you will not be in the best position to discover the real reasons for what happened. If a friend of yours was in this situation, how would you explain what had happened? How many possible reasons can you think of? If you remain open-minded and ask yourself what other explanations there might be, you may discover that what happened might have had absolutely nothing to do with you.

Am I expecting myself to be perfect?

If this is something that often comes up for you, it could reflect one of your Rules for Living. As we have said, people with low self-esteem often expect a great deal of themselves. But it is just not possible to get everything 100 per cent right all the time. If you expect to do so, you are inevitably setting yourself up to fail. Accepting that you aren't perfect means setting realistic targets for yourself, and giving yourself credit when you reach them, even if you haven't achieved perfection. This will encourage you to feel better about yourself, and so motivate you to keep going and try again. It also means that you can learn from your difficulties and mistakes, rather than being upset and even paralysed by them.

5 What can I do?

How can I put a new, kinder perspective into practice?

Here's where we come once again to the importance of direct experience – experiments. How can you find out if your alternative perspective works better for you? Is there anything you can do to change the situation that sparked the self-critical thoughts (e.g.

changing or leaving a job where you are not valued, or ending a relationship with a person who reinforces your negative view of yourself)? Or could you change your own reactions? Old habits die hard – what will you do in future if you find yourself thinking, feeling and acting in the same old way? How would you like to handle the situation differently, next time it occurs?

One helpful possibility is to ask yourself: how would someone who truly believed my new alternative behave? What would they do differently? And what if *I* experimented with behaving the same way, even if I am not yet fully convinced that my alternatives are true? Here is your opportunity systematically to experiment with behaving in new ways that are less self-defeating, kinder and more compassionate (e.g. accepting compliments gracefully, not apologising for yourself, taking opportunities, asserting your own needs, etc.). Record your ideas on the chart, and then take every opportunity to try them out, to develop and strengthen a new, fair, healthy perspective on yourself. We shall return to this in more detail in Section 3.

SUMMARY

1. Self-critical thoughts are triggered when you sense that an event or experience has confirmed your Bottom Line.
2. Self-critical thinking is a learned habit. It does not necessarily reflect the truth about you.
3. Self-criticism does more harm than good. Believing your self-critical thoughts makes you feel bad and encourages you to act in self-defeating ways.
4. You can learn to stand back from self-critical thoughts and see them simply as the voice of low self-esteem speaking – something you automatically do, rather than as a reflection of your true self.

---

5. Self-critical thoughts, like anxious predictions, can be questioned. You can observe them and their impact on your feelings, body state and behaviour, and then re-think them and search for more balanced and kindly perspectives on yourself.

6. The final step is to experiment with acting differently, treating yourself more fairly and kindly, valuing your strengths, qualities, assets and talents as you would those of another person you cared about. This will be our focus in the next section.

SECTION 3:

Learning to Accept and Appreciate Your Positive Qualities

In Sections 1 and 2 of this part of the handbook, you learned how to check out anxious predictions and question self-critical thoughts. These skills are vital in establishing a new, fairer and more balanced Bottom Line (central belief about yourself). In Section 3, we shall look at the other side of the coin – becoming more aware of your personal qualities and resources, talents and strengths, and learning to treat yourself with respect and consideration. Changing the negative biases in how you see yourself to a more balanced perspective is not always quick and easy. If you learned to think badly of yourself at an early age, you will not have developed a habit of accepting and appreciating yourself as you are. If this is the case, then be aware that change may take time. Be persistent, and keep an open mind, so that you can take advantage of the methods described here to move further towards healthy self-esteem – the sense that it is OK to be exactly who you are.

This section will help you understand:

- how to develop a balanced view of yourself
- how to identify your good points and positive qualities
- how to make them real
- how to value everyday pleasures and achievements

- how to treat yourself with respect and kindness, and increase your enjoyment of the good things in your life

Try this exercise.

How would you react to hearing someone make the following statements?

- 'I'm beautiful'
- 'I'm clever'
- 'I'm a brilliant cook'
- 'I have a terrific sense of humour'
- 'I am a gifted musician'
- 'I'm adorable'
- 'I'm great'

Tick your most likely reactions. Would you:

☐ a. Be delighted to meet someone so gifted?
☐ b. Feel uncomfortable and disapproving?
☐ c. Find yourself muttering 'Bighead', or 'Talk about blowing your own trumpet'?
☐ d. Instantly take it for granted that these things must be true?
☐ e. See such statements as boasting, getting above oneself?
☐ f. Feel that it was about time this person was cut down to size?

If you have low self-esteem, you may well have ticked b, c, e and f. The idea of allowing yourself to acknowledge your good points may seem to you like boasting. The very thought may make you squirm with embarrassment. You may also fear that, if you admit anything good about yourself, someone else will be sure to step in and say 'Oh, no, you aren't'. Such feelings stand in the way of healthy self-esteem.

Yet, in fact, the idea that self-acceptance – noticing and taking pleasure in your strengths and qualities, treating yourself with care and consideration, and allowing yourself to enjoy and savour the good things in your life – will inevitably lead to smugness and complacency makes no sense. Self-acceptance (that is, a clear-eyed, realistic assessment of your strong points alongside your natural human weaknesses) is part of healthy self-esteem, not self-inflation. In fact, ignoring your positive qualities helps to keep low self-esteem going, because it stops you from having a balanced view that takes into account the good things about yourself as well as your genuine shortcomings and things you might prefer to change.

In this section, you have an opportunity to try out two main strategies for self-acceptance, using the three core skills you have already practised (awareness, re-thinking and experiments). The first strategy is to bring your positive qualities into focus, to learn to accept the good things about yourself. The second is to learn to feel worthy of treating yourself with the same respect and consideration you would give to another person you cared for, allowing yourself to experience fully life's pleasures and to give yourself credit for what you do. In essence, you are learning to be a good friend to yourself, to value and appreciate yourself, just as you are.

Bringing your good qualities into focus (Awareness)

Learning to acknowledge and value your good qualities involves three steps:

1. Recognising
2. Reliving
3. Recording

We shall look at each of these in turn.

Step 1: Recognising

It is impossible to value your good points if you have no idea what they are. So, the first step to a balanced view is simply to learn to recognise them and bring them into focus, rather than letting them pass you by. A helpful starting point is to make a list of your qualities, talents, skills and strengths. As well as enhancing your self-esteem, this will sharpen your awareness of how you discount and ignore your good points – you will see something that keeps you stuck in low self-esteem *as it actually happens.*

As you embark on this task, be on the alert for self-critical thoughts – they are almost certain to pop up when you start to focus on your good qualities. To begin with, you will probably not be able to stop them from automatically popping into your mind, but you can learn to take them less seriously. Your aim is to be able to notice these 'yes, buts' calmly ('Oh, look, there's another one') and let them go, rather than feeling you need to believe them, feel bad about them, or act on them. They will weaken and decay, once you can see them for what they are and refuse to let them get in your way. If you can do so, simply put them to one side and continue with your task. If on the other hand they keep competing for your attention and are hard to dismiss, then record them on a **Questioning Self-Critical Thoughts Chart** (see Section 2, p. 158) and find answers to them before moving on.

IT'S WORTH REMEMBERING . . .

Self-criticism is a habit that will weaken, so long as you keep self-critical thoughts in perspective and refuse to allow them to stop you adopting a more balanced view of yourself.

Some people find making a list of positive qualities quite easy. Their doubts about themselves may be relatively weak or may surface only in particularly challenging situations. Other people, with very powerful and convincing Bottom Lines, find listing positive qualities almost impossible. The habit of screening them out and discounting them can be so strong that it is difficult at first to accept any good points at all. Most people are somewhere in between.

You may find that you need some help, perhaps from a close friend or someone else you care about and trust. It is worth investing your time in this task. Even if it takes a while to come up with a good list, becoming aware of your positive qualities as part of everyday living will eventually have a considerable impact on how you feel about yourself.

In order to get started:

- Choose a time and place where you can be sure you will not be interrupted and settle down to make your list.
- Make sure you are sitting somewhere comfortable, where you feel peaceful and relaxed. You could perhaps put on some music you enjoy.
- Now, in the box on p. 190, make a list of as many good things about yourself as you can think of. You may be able to list several straight away. Or you may be hard put to think of even one or two. You can use the questions below to help you if you wish.
- Give yourself plenty of time, and don't worry if the task is hard at first. You are trying something new, finding a fresh perspective on yourself.
- Take your list as far as you can, and when you feel you have come up with as many items as possible for the time being, stop.
- Put your list somewhere easily accessible – it may even be helpful to carry it with you. Over the next few days, even if you are not actually working on it, keep it at the back of your mind and add to it as things occur to you.
- Be pleased even if you can find only one or two things to begin with. You have made a good start in freeing up your thinking and taken the first crucial step towards acknowledging and accepting good things about yourself.

MY GOOD POINTS (qualities, talents, skills, strengths)

How to identify your good points and positive qualities

If your self-esteem has been low for some time, you will almost certainly have difficulty in identifying your strong points and positive qualities. This does not mean that you do not have any – it just means that you are out of the habit of noticing and appreciating them. Here are some questions to help you. Notice that each question is picking up on a possible 'yes, but', for example, 'Yes, but it's only small', 'Yes, but I'm not always like that', 'Yes, but other people are more like that than I am', and so on.

KEY QUESTIONS

To Help You Identify Your Good Points

1. What do you like about yourself, however small and fleeting?
2. What positive qualities do you possess?
3. What have you achieved in your life, however small?
4. What challenges have you faced in your life?
5. What gifts or talents do you have, however modest?
6. What skills have you acquired?
7. What do other people like or value in you?
8. What qualities and actions that you value in others do you share?
9. What aspects of yourself would you appreciate if they were aspects of another person?
10. What small positives are you discounting?
11. What are the bad qualities you do *not* have?
12. How might another person who cared about you describe you?

---

1 *What do you like about yourself, however small and fleeting?*

- Look out for anything about yourself that you have ever felt able to appreciate, even if only for a moment.

2 *What positive qualities do you possess?*

- Include qualities that you feel you do not possess 100 per cent, or that you do not show all the time.
- Give yourself credit for having the quality at all, rather than discounting it because you have it to a less than perfect extent.

3 What have you achieved in your life, however small?

- You are not looking for anything earth-shattering here – like winning the Olympics or being the first to cross the Sahara on a donkey.
- Take into account small successes, small steps you have successfully achieved.

4 What challenges have you faced in your life?

- What anxieties and problems have you tried to conquer?
- What difficulties have you dealt with?
- What qualities in you do these efforts reflect?
- Facing challenges and anxieties takes courage and persistence, whether or not you resolve them successfully. Give yourself credit for this.
- And don't forget the challenge you are facing right now – the challenge of overcoming your low self-esteem. Give yourself credit for all these things.

5 What gifts or talents do you have, however modest?

- What do you do well? (Take note: '*well*', not 'perfectly'!)
- Again, remember to include the small things. You do not need to be Michelangelo or Beethoven. If you can boil an egg, or whistle a tune, or make someone laugh, then add it to the list.

6 What skills have you acquired?

- What do you know how to do? Include work skills, domestic skills, people skills, academic skills, sporting skills and leisure skills.
- For example, do you know how to use a smartphone, a computer, a microwave or a saw?

- Can you catch a ball? Can you drive a car or ride a bicycle? Do you know how to swim, how to sew or how to clean a bathroom?
- Are you good at listening to people, or appreciating their jokes? Can you read in a thoughtful way? Have you learned any languages?
- Think about all the different areas of your life and note down skills you have in all of them, however partial or basic.

7 What do other people like or value in you?

- What do they thank you for, ask you to do, or compliment you on?
- What do they praise or appreciate?
- You may not have been paying much attention to this. Now is the time to start.

8 What qualities and actions that you value in other people do you share?

- It may be easier for you to see other people's strong points than your own. Which positive qualities that you appreciate in others do you also possess?
- Beware of unfavourable comparisons here. You do not have to be or do whatever it is to the same degree as the other person. You just need to acknowledge that you share the quality, even if only to a more limited extent.

9 What aspects of yourself would you appreciate if they were aspects of another person?

- If there are aspects of yourself that you would appreciate if they were another person's, write them on your list.
- Think also about things you do that you would appreciate and value if another person did them.

- Write down anything that you would count as a positive if it were done by someone else.

10 What small positives are you discounting?

- You may feel that you should only include major positives on your list. But would you discount small negatives in the same way?
- If not, write the small positives down. Otherwise it will be impossible to achieve a balanced view.

11 What are the bad qualities you do not have?

- Think of some bad qualities (e.g. 'irresponsible', 'cruel' or 'dishonest'). Is this how you would describe yourself?
- If your answer is 'no', then you must be something else. What is it (e.g. 'responsible', 'kind' or 'honest')?
- Write down the mirror images of the bad qualities you identified. Again, don't discount the good qualities because you don't think you possess them to a great enough extent.

12 How might another person who cared about you describe you?

- Think about someone you know who cares about you, respects you and is on your side. They may have a more balanced view of you than you have of yourself.
- What sort of person would they say you were? What words or phrases would they use to describe you? How would they see you as a friend, a parent, a colleague or a member of your community?
- If there is someone close to you, whom you respect and trust, ask them to make a list of the things they like and value in you. Choose someone you have good reason to believe cares

about you and wishes you well (e.g. a parent, a brother or sister, a partner, a child, a friend or a colleague with whom you have a close relationship). You may find their list a very pleasant surprise, and it will strengthen your relationship.

• Again, watch out for thoughts that lead you to discount and devalue what you read (for example, that they are only doing it to be kind and can't possibly mean what they say). If you have thoughts like these, write them down and answer them on a **Questioning Self-Critical Thoughts Chart** (see Section 2, p. 158).

MAKING A LIST OF YOUR GOOD POINTS: LIN'S STORY

Lin, the artist described in Part One of the course whose parents had never been able to appreciate her talent, had some difficulty with her list, as you might imagine. Experience had taught her to place very little value on herself, and in particular to devalue what to other people appeared a striking gift. At first, she could not think of anything to write except 'good-natured' and 'hard-working'. Trying to add other items roused all sorts of reservations (e.g. 'But other people are better at that than me' or 'But that isn't really important').

After a couple of tries, she used the questions on p. 191 to free up her thinking. She still found it hard but eventually added 'thoughtful', 'practical', 'good colour sense', 'persistent', 'creative', 'kind', 'good taste', 'adventurous cook' and 'open to new ideas'. In addition, she screwed up her courage and asked an old and trusted friend if he would make a list of her good points too. He said it was about time she gave her confidence a boost and set to with a will. Lin was moved and delighted by the affection that shone through his list. He echoed some of the items on her own list, and added 'makes me laugh', 'good listener', 'good drinking companion', 'has created a welcoming home', 'intelligent', 'sensitive' and 'warm'.

Step 2: Reliving

Once you have begun recognising your good qualities, the next step is to help them to sink in, to make them real. On its own, a list is a good first step – but it is not enough. Your list will be most helpful to you if you use it as a basis for raising your awareness of your good qualities, aiming for the point where recognising, acknowledging and valuing them has become second nature, and where accepting them becomes something you can feel on a gut level, rather than something theoretical which you can easily ignore or forget. Of course, this will not happen overnight. You will need to practise deliberately directing attention to them. One way of doing this is to call up vivid memories of times when you have demonstrated them in what you did.

Give yourself a few days to notice more items to add to your list and then, when you feel you have taken it as far as you can for the time being, once again find yourself a comfortable, relaxing spot and read the list to yourself.

Pause and dwell on each good point and quality you have recorded, and let it sink in. When you have read slowly and carefully through the list, go back to the top again. Now, as you consider each item, bring to mind a particular time when you showed that quality in your actions. Take time to make the memory as clear and vivid as you can. Close your eyes, relax, and recall it in detail – almost as if you were living it again:

- When was it?
- Where were you?
- Who were you with?
- What exactly did you do that showed this quality in action?
- Try to tune in to your senses. What could you see, at the time? And hear? What about sensations in your body – taste, touch, smell, your sense of your body position?
- And see if you can call up the emotions you experienced at the time,

- Finally, what were the consequences of what you did (what did you notice, how did you feel, how did others react, and so on)?

Notice what effect this exercise has on your mood and how you feel about yourself. If you can absorb yourself in it fully, recreating what happened in your mind's eye and calling up the feelings you had at the time, you will find that the items on your list become much more vivid and meaningful to you. You should find your mood lifting, and you may begin to notice a growing sense of self-acceptance and confidence.

If this does not happen, look out for feelings of shame, embarrassment or disbelief. These feelings may indicate the presence of self-critical thoughts. Are you, for example, telling yourself that it is wrong to be so smug? Do you feel as if you are showing off? Are you thinking that what you did was trivial – anyone could have done it? Are you telling yourself that you could have done it better? Or faster? Or more effectively? Or are you devaluing your qualities because you think they are too ordinary to be worth considering?

When 'yes, buts' like these intrude, simply notice their presence and put them to one side. Then go back to focusing fully on your list of positive qualities. Remember: it takes time for these old habits to die away, so there is no need to worry if you find them turning up again. If they are too strong to be easily put aside, you can tackle them by using the skills you learned for dealing with self-critical thoughts in Section 2.

Step 3: Recording

The next step is to make awareness of your good qualities an everyday event. A good way to do this is by recording examples every day on a **Good Points Chart**, as they occur, just as you previously recorded examples of anxious predictions and self-critical thoughts.

Your objective is to reach the point where you automatically notice examples of your good qualities, without needing any reminder or record. You may reach this point in a few weeks, or it may take longer – give it whatever time it needs. Once you get there, there is no further need for the record, though in fact you may like to continue, and it may also be helpful to return to recording if something happens to give your confidence a knock.

Use your list of qualities, skills, strengths and talents as a prompt to help you get started and keep a copy of your **Chart** with you, so that you can record things *as soon as they happen*. Otherwise, examples may be missed, forgotten or discounted. Decide in advance how many examples of good qualities you wish to record every day. Many people find that three is about right to start with. If this seems to be too many, however, then don't be afraid to start with two, or even one. Wherever you start, as you get into the swing of it, you will be able to add more. When recording three incidents is easy, increase the number to four. When four is easy, go up to five, and so on. By then, noticing pluses should be pretty automatic.

For each entry on the chart, record the date and time, a description of what you did, and what good quality it showed. Make sure that what you did and the circumstances in which you did it are described in enough detail for you to remember what it was when you look back on it, e.g. 'helped old Mrs Jackson cross the road with her shopping', not 'was kind'.

On the opposite page is an example of a **Good Points Chart,** filled in by Lin. Notice that she does not just record 'hard-working', 'funny', 'kind' and so on on her chart. There is enough detail for her to be able to remember later what happened. So, the record can be a resource for her, to reflect on, to reinforce her new perspective on herself, and to call on at times of difficulty.

On pages 200–202 you will find **Good Points Charts** for you to fill in. There are two other blank charts at the back of the handbook, which you can photocopy if you wish, or you can download them from www.overcoming.co.uk.

Good Points Chart: Lin		
Date/Time	**What I did**	**Positive quality**
12 March morning	Spent several hours completing a large landscape painting	Hard-working
12 March evening	Went out with Simon. Haven't laughed so much in ages	Good drinking companion, funny
13 March afternoon	Bought flowers	Creating a welcoming home
13 March evening	Tried cooking a Thai curry for the first time — tasted odd, but was edible	Adventurous cook
14 March morning	Called Mother as it was her birthday	Kind
14 March afternoon	Fixed shelving in workroom	Practical

Good Points Chart		
Date/Time	What I did	Positive quality

Good Points Chart		
Date/Time	What I did	Positive quality

Good Points Chart		
Date/Time	What I did	Positive quality

At the end of each day, perhaps just before you go to bed, make time to relax and be comfortable and review your chart. Look over what you have recorded and recreate the memory of what you did in vivid detail. Let it sink in, so that it affects your feelings and your sense of yourself. You can also review your charts at the end of the week, to get an overview, and to decide how many examples of good points to look out for the following week. They will become a store of pleasure, confidence-building memories that you can call on any time you are feeling stressed, low or bad about yourself.

Treating yourself with respect, consideration and kindness

As well as failing to notice or value their good points, people with low self-esteem often miss out on the richness of everyday experience in two major ways. They do not make any effort to make life pleasurable and satisfying, and they do not give themselves credit for what they do. This is especially likely to happen when you are feeling down or depressed, and it helps to keep you stuck in low self-esteem.

The first step towards learning to value your everyday experiences is to get a clear picture of how you spend your time, how satisfying your pattern of daily activities is to you, and how good you are at acknowledging your achievements and successes (awareness). You can use what you discover as a jumping-off point for change (experiments). And once again you may well encounter self-defeating thoughts as you go about this, and you can use your re-thinking skills to tackle them.

Increasing pleasure and satisfaction: The 'Daily Activity Diary' (DAD)

The **Daily Activity Diary (DAD)** is one way of getting the information you need. You will find an example filled in by Lin on pp. 205–208, followed by blank sheets to use for yourself if you wish. There are more at the end of the book, and at www.overcoming.co.uk.

The diary looks a bit like a school timetable, with the days across the top and the times down the left-hand side – but don't let that put you off! It will give you a real insight into how you spend your time and a basis for finding a pattern of activity that really works for you. Each day is divided into hourly slots, in which you can record what you do and what you gain from what you do. This means noting how much you enjoy your activities (Pleasure – P) and how far you give yourself credit for your achievements (Achievement – A).

The **DAD** can help you to:

- keep an accurate record of your everyday experiences, as they happen
- identify changes you would like to make in how you spend your time
- focus on positive aspects of your experience (just as you have been learning to focus on positive aspects of yourself)
- spot 'killjoy thoughts' that lead you to discount and disqualify your pleasures and successes

Daily Activity Diary: Lin

	Monday	Tuesday	Wednesday	Thursday	Friday	Saturday	Sunday
6–7				Sleep	Sleep	Sleep	Sleep
7–8				"	" AO P3	"	"
8–9				" AO P5	Got up; coffee; shower A3 P2	"	AO P5
9–10				Got up; breakfast; radio A1 P4	Out to buy art materials	" AO P5	Got up – tired; breakfast; shower A5 P2
10–11				Worked A2 P4	" A3 P4	Got up; breakfast; shower A2 P4	Worked A5 P2
11–12				" A2 P6	Coffee with M. AO P6	Drove out to Henley A3 P4	" A4 P5

MORNING

Daily Activity Diary: Lin continued

	Monday	Tuesday	Wednesday	Thursday	Friday	Saturday	Sunday
AFTERNOON							
12–1				" A1 P6	Worked A6 P3	Lunch with cousins A1 P6	" A4 P5
1–2			Met agent for L. wants me to exhibit A5 P0	Lunch in park AO P6	" A6 P5	"	Lunch with J. AO P6
2–3			" A4 P1	Cleaned up mess in apartment A7 P0	" A4 P7	"	AO P8
3–4			Went round to see F. AO P1	" A8 P0	Called agent and agreed to exhibit A10 P2	Walked along the river by myself A2 P5	Went to the zoo with J. AO P8
4–5			" AO P5	Sat & read A1 P4	Worked A4 P6	A3 P5	"

EVENING

5–6	Home AO P2	" A8 P3	" A4 P6	Shopping A2 P3	Worked A6 P3
6–7	Worked A2 P4	Drove home A3 P2	" A3 P1	met J. & F. for drinks & eats A1 P6	" A4 P6
7–8	" A5 P2	Phoned Mum A4 P1	Supper A1 P4	Theatre AO P10	Supper A1 P4
8–9	" A3 P4	Listened to music, thinking about work	TV AO P6	"	P. came round depressed A4 P2
9–10	" A2 P6	" AO P6	" AO P8	"	" A4 P4
10–11	Bed AO P5	Met P. for late drink A1 P7	" AO P1	Pub again AO P8	Read AO P6
11–12	"	"	Bed AO P4	Back to J's apartment AO P8	Bed AO P4
12–1	"	Bed AO P8!	"	"	"

Review: (What do you notice about your day? What worked for you? What did not work? What would you like to change?)

Mon:

Tues:

Weds: Didn't enjoy lunch at all. He was hassling me. As usual, couldn't believe anyone would really like my work.

Thurs: Some good work, which I enjoyed. Great evening – worth planning more of this.

Fri: Hard to get started on work but sticking with it paid off. Called agent and said yes – terrifying but I need to do it. Treated myself to relaxed, mindless evening at home.

Sat: Walk a good idea but too long. Should have paced myself.

Sun: Planned lunch w. J a great success. Lot of fun watching street theatre in Covent Garden.

Over the course of a week or so, keep a detailed daily record of your activities, hour by hour. You will gather the most useful information if the week you record is typical of your life at the moment. This is the information that will be most helpful when you come to consider changes you wish to make. If you record your activities over an exceptional week (e.g. you were on holiday, you were off work sick, or your mother had come to stay), the information you gather will only really be directly relevant to similar times in the future, not to your everyday life.

Each hour, record:

What you did

Simply note the activity (or activities) you were engaged in. Anything you do counts as an activity, including sleeping and doing nothing in particular. Even 'doing nothing' is actually doing something. What does it mean exactly? Sitting, staring into space? Pottering around, doing minor domestic tasks? Sitting slumped on the couch, channel-surfing?

Rating of Pleasure (P)

How much did you enjoy what you did? Give each activity a rating between 0 and 10 for Pleasure (P). 'P10' would mean you enjoyed it very, very much. Lin, for example, gave 'P10' to Thursday's evening at the theatre with friends. She felt she had thoroughly enjoyed herself. The play was excellent, funny and thought-provoking, and she had had a really good time with people she knew very well and felt completely relaxed with. 'P5' would mean moderate enjoyment. So, for example, Lin gave 'P5' to Saturday's walk in the country by herself. She had enjoyed the warmth of the sunny day, but had miscalculated the distance, so that she was very tired by the time she got back to her car. 'P0' would mean you did not enjoy an activity at all. Lin gave 'P0' to Wednesday's meeting with her agent, who was hassling her to exhibit her recent paintings – even though normally she would have enjoyed his company as she liked and respected him.

You can use any number between 0 and 10 to show how much you enjoyed a particular activity. Like Lin, you will probably find that your pleasure level varies, according to what you do. This variation will be a useful source of information. It shows what works for you, and what does not work. It may give you clues about killjoy thoughts that get in the way of satisfaction and enjoyment. (For example, Lin was aware that she could not enjoy talking to her agent because she was preoccupied with fears about exposing her work to public view.)

Rating of Achievement (A)

How far was each activity an experience of mastering something that took effort? This is what we mean by achievement here. These activities may not in themselves be wildly pleasurable, but they give you a sense of taking care of business, acting in your own best interests, doing things that need to be done – in short, taking control of your life rather than allowing it to take control of you.

'A10' would mean a very considerable achievement. Lin gave herself 'A10' for the phone call she made to her agent on Friday. This was because she called to agree that she would submit work to an exhibition, despite her anxieties. She gave herself a high 'A' rating as recognition that this was a difficult thing to do, and she had to push herself, but she did it. 'A5' would mean a moderate achievement. Lin gave herself 'A5' on Sunday morning when she got up in time to complete a picture she was working on, despite still feeling tired from her walk. Her first reaction was that getting up was nothing special, but she realised on reflection that, given how tired she felt, it was quite an achievement. 'A0' would mean no sort of achievement at all. Lin gave herself 'A0' for an evening at home watching television. This was pure self-indulgence, and she enjoyed it, but it did not involve any sort of achievement and so she felt happy to give it a 0 for 'A'.

Again, like Lin, you could use any number between 0 and 10 to judge how much achievement was involved in carrying out a particular activity.

It is important to realise that 'achievement' as we use it here does not only refer to major achievements like getting a promotion, hosting a party for a hundred guests, or spring-cleaning the whole house from top to bottom. Nor does it only mean things you have done really, really well. Everyday activities can be real achievements, for which you deserve to give yourself credit. This is especially the case if you are feeling stressed, tired, unwell or depressed. When you are not in a good state emotionally, even relatively minor routine activities (answering the telephone, making a snack, getting to work on time, even getting out of bed) can represent substantial achievements. Not recognising this often leads people with low self-esteem to devalue what they do and, of course, this helps to keep low self-esteem going.

So, when you rate 'A', remember to take into account how you felt at the time. Ask yourself: 'How much of an achievement was this activity, *given how I felt at the time?*' If carrying out the activity represents a triumph over feeling bad, a real effort, a difficulty confronted, then you deserve to give yourself credit for it, even if it was routine, not done to your usual standard, or not completed.

Finding a balance that works for you

Make sure that you rate all your activities for both P and A. Some activities (e.g. duties, obligations, tasks) are mainly A activities. Others are mainly P (relaxing and pleasurable things that we do just for ourselves). Many activities are a mixture of the two. For example, going to a party might warrant a good A rating if socialising makes you anxious, because it represents a triumph over your negative predictions. But once you arrived and began to relax and have a good time, the party could become enjoyable, too. In the long run, you are aiming for a balance of A and P. Giving both ratings to all your activities will help you to find this balance.

Review

At the end of each day, take a few minutes to look back over your diary. A brief daily review will encourage you to reflect on what you have done, rather than simply recording it and leaving it.

- What do you notice about your day?
- What does the record tell you about how you are spending your time, and how much pleasure and satisfaction you get from what you do?
- How easy was it to give yourself credit for your achievements?
- What worked for you?
- What did not work?
- What were the high points, both in terms of pleasure and of achievement?
- What were the low points?
- What would you like more of or less of?
- What changes would you like to make?

Now is your chance to fill in your own **Daily Activity Diary**. You will find copies on pp. 216 and more blank diary sheets, which you can photocopy if you wish, on pp. 434 or online. The first four are for recording what you do now, as we have just described. The rest are for the next step: planning your day so as to maximise your enjoyment and satisfaction in what you do.

Frequently asked questions about filling in the Daily Activity Diary

Here are some questions people often ask about the Daily Activity Diary (DAD).

How long should I carry on keeping the record?

The objective of the record is to give you a clear idea of how you are spending your time, and how pleasurable and satisfying your daily activities are to you. The record is also an opportunity to start noticing how negative thinking patterns (e.g. anxious predictions or self-critical thoughts) may prevent you from making the most of your experiences. So, continue the record until you feel you have enough information for these objectives to be met. For many people, a week or two is enough. But if you feel you need more time to hone your awareness, then there is no need to stop at that point.

When should I complete the record sheet?

Just as with the other worksheets you have used, it is important to record what you did, and your ratings, *at the time*, whenever possible. If it's not possible for some reason to use the DAD itself, make a quick note on anything that comes to hand. You can transfer your record to the chart later on. It is worth doing this because, in the course of a busy day, things are easily forgotten. In addition, negative biases are likely to give you a clear memory of things that did not go well, and to screen out pleasures, successes and achievements (especially if you are feeling generally low and bad about yourself). Noting your activities and ratings *at the time* will help to counter this bias. Immediate ratings will also help you to tune in to even small pleasures and achievements that may otherwise go unnoticed. Finally, if you put off recording what you do, you are more likely to forget to do it, put it off until tomorrow, or perhaps give up altogether before you have collected the information you need.

What if I discover that I am not enjoying anything very much?

This could be because you are not making space in your day for enjoyable activities. Perhaps you are genuinely very busy dealing with a range of responsibilities (e.g. work or study pressures, the needs of your family, looking after elderly parents, your commitment to a neighbourhood network or charity) and giving yourself pleasurable and relaxing 'me time' simply falls off the bottom of your 'to do' list. You can use the **DAD** to check whether this is so, and then work out ways of ensuring that your day includes activities that will relax you and replenish your resources. Even small pauses and moments of pleasure (an extra couple of minutes in the shower, lingering over a coffee, pausing to notice what is around you as you walk to work) will make a difference if you approach them as precious breathing spaces, opportunities to refresh and energise yourself.

Or perhaps you have a Rule that makes you uncomfortable with putting yourself first or taking time out to do things you enjoy. It feels selfish to prioritise your own needs in this way. If you suspect that this may be the case, look carefully at the pattern of your day. How much time is given over to activities which are pleasurable, relaxing, fun and just for you? Remember: if your day is filled with tasks, obligations, duties and things you do for others, you may end up feeling drained and resentful – exactly the opposite of your generous intentions. Maybe at the next stage you could experiment with introducing more enjoyable activities into your day.

Or perhaps you do not feel you deserve to enjoy yourself – you are not good enough. Lin, for example, became aware by keeping the record that, once she had committed herself to a particular piece of work, she did not feel entitled to make time for pleasurable activities until she had completed it and it had been approved.

On the other hand, maybe you are engaging in activities that should be pleasurable, but killjoy thoughts are preventing you from enjoying them fully. Your record could help you to tune in to this. Look for examples in your record of activities that should have been enjoyable, but in fact were not. Ask yourself:

- What was going on while you were engaging in them?
- Were you fully absorbed in what you were doing? Or were you actually preoccupied with other things?
- Were you making comparisons with other people, who seem to be enjoying themselves more than you?
- Were you making comparisons with how things used to be at some time in the past, or with how you think things *should* be?

(Frequently asked questions continue on p. 220.)

Daily Activity Diary		Monday	Tuesday	Wednesday	Thursday	Friday	Saturday	Sunday
MORNING	6–7							
	7–8							
	8–9							
	9–10							
	10–11							
	11–12							

12-1	1-2	2-3	3-4	4-5
A F T E R N O O N				

	Monday	Tuesday	Wednesday	Thursday	Friday	Saturday	Sunday
5–6							
6–7							
7–8							
8–9							
9–10							
10–11							

EVENING

11–12		
12–1		

Review: (What do you notice about your day? What worked for you? What did not work? What would you like to change?)

Mon:

Tues:

Weds:

Thurs:

Fri:

Sat:

Sun:

If, when you engage in potentially pleasurable activities, your mind is actually elsewhere, then you will not enjoy them. So, watch out for killjoy thoughts and, practise putting them to one side ('Ah, there you are again!') and absorbing yourself in what you are doing, engaging all your senses to the full. If the thoughts are too strong to put to one side, then write them down and look for alternatives to them (re-thinking) just as you did with anxious predictions and self-critical thoughts. This is the beauty of the core skills you are learning: they can be used with any painful and unhelpful thoughts that upset you and get in the way of leading the life you long to lead.

There is one other possibility, if you find that you are not really enjoying anything at all as you used to. This is one of the classic signs of depression. So, look back at the signs of depression described on p. 5. If this picture fits you, you may need to seek treatment for depression in its own right. A good starting point might be to read Paul Gilbert's book in the 'Overcoming' series, *Overcoming Depression*, or perhaps consult *The Complete CBT Guide for Depression and Low Mood* (also an 'Overcoming' publication).

What if I'm not achieving anything?

If this appears to be the case, use your record to find out more about what is going on. Perhaps anxious predictions and self-critical thoughts are leading you to restrict your field of activities.

- Do you miss opportunities, for example out of anxiety that you will not be able to cope with them?
- Do you avoid social contacts, in case you make a fool of yourself, or people reject you?
- Do you avoid challenges, convinced that you will not be able to meet them?

If so, then continuing to work on your anxious and self-critical thoughts should help you extend your range of activities, which will allow you to gain a more positive view of your capabilities and enhance your sense of achievement.

If on the other hand you already engage in a wide range of activities, including some that are quite difficult or challenging, perhaps you are allowing self-critical thinking to undermine your sense of achievement. Self-critical thinking reduces motivation and gives a false impression that you are achieving nothing. It may well be based on very high standards you have for yourself (your Rules for Living). Perhaps these prevent you from acknowledging small successes because you think they are not special enough, or should have been done better or faster or more completely?

Watch what runs through your mind when you complete a task. Do your thoughts make you feel good and motivate you to do more? Or do they demoralise and discourage you and leave you feeling you did not do very well and there's little point in continuing? If so, you need to write them down and re-think them, using the skills you have already acquired. Treating yourself more kindly, giving yourself credit, and encouraging yourself will take you further than downgrading what you do and putting yourself down.

How can you increase your enjoyment of life? (Experiments)

Once you have seen how you spend your time, the next step is to introduce changes that will increase your enjoyment, enhance your sense of pleasure and achievement, and so help you to feel better about yourself.

Your daily review of your diary should already have given you some idea of the changes you might like to make. Now you can start planning ahead so as to create a balance between *Achievement* activities (duties, challenges, obligations, tasks) and *Pleasure* activities (relaxation, enjoyment). Planning ahead is a commitment to yourself, a statement that you intend to take this seriously, that you value your time and want to make the most of each day.

As a starting point, think about what you are going to do today – or tomorrow, if this is evening time. Then write down three activities that might give you *Pleasure*:

1. _____

2. _____

3. _____

And now three activities that might give you a sense of *Achievement*, for example tasks that you have been putting off or avoiding:

1. _____

2. _____

3. _____

Now decide how to fit these activities into your day. When exactly will you do each of them, and for how long? Write this down alongside each activity.

Planning your day

There are a number of things you will need to do, each one a step towards a more satisfying and enjoyable life. Details about each one start on the next page. In order to plan each day systematically, using the **DAD**s at the back of the book on pp. 434–443, you will need to:

Write down your plan for the day

You may prefer to do this first thing in the morning, or in the evening. Choose whichever time is likely to be easiest for you. For example, if your morning is usually madly busy, you could do without the extra task. Use the evening (perhaps when you are relaxing just before going to bed) instead. If, on the other hand, you are normally too tired in the evening to think straight, but usually wake feeling refreshed, then use the morning. You can record your plan in draft on the **DAD** itself, if you wish, or somewhere completely separate if you prefer.

Each day aim for a balance between *Pleasure* and *Achievement*. If you fill your time with duties and chores, and allow no time for enjoyment, you may end up tired and resentful. On the other hand, if you completely ignore things you have to do, you may find your enjoyment soured by a sense that nothing has been achieved, and the list of tasks you are putting off will keep hanging about at the back of your mind making it difficult to really enjoy anything.

Record what you actually do

Use your plan as a guide for the day and record what you actually do on the **DAD**. Rate each activity from 0 to 10 for *Pleasure* and *Achievement*, just as you did at the self-observation stage.

REVIEW YOUR DAY

At the end of each day, take a few minutes to sit down comfortably, relax, and review what you have done. Thoughtfully examine how you spent your time:

- How far did you stick to your plan?
- If you did not, why was that?
- Did you get sidetracked?

- Did something come up that you had not predicted?
- Had you planned too much to start with?
- How much enjoyment and satisfaction did you get from what you did?
- How good was your balance between *P* and *A*?
- What would you like more of or less of?
- What would you like to change?
- What was the impact of your pattern of activities on your mood and how you feel about yourself?

Once you get the hang of planning ahead, you may well find that you are automatically looking after yourself by balancing out *Achievement* and *Pleasure* without needing to record anything. However, a written plan may still be helpful at times in the future, e.g. when you are feeling low and finding it difficult to motivate yourself, or when you are under pressure and need to be reminded that being busy doesn't have to exclude all pleasure and relaxation.

Frequently asked questions about planning ahead

Here are some questions people often ask about planning the day so as to maximise *Pleasure* and sense of *Achievement*.

What if my plan is a success?

Success means devising a realistic plan, with a good balance of pleasurable activities and achievements, accomplishing what you set out to do, and getting the enjoyment and sense of mastery you wanted. If your plan works for you in this way, you have something really positive to build on. You have clearly found a pattern to the day which works well for you, and which you will want to repeat.

However, even if your plan is generally successful, you may still find it helpful to carry out some fine-tuning. For example, you might want to add some regular exercise, or some quality time with your family. Or you might decide to contact someone you have lost touch with, or to tackle a particular task you have been putting off.

What if my plan doesn't work out?

Plans fail to work out for many reasons. In fact, if you look closely at what happened, this is likely to be very useful, because it may tell you why your pattern of activity is not working for you. Here is a chance to find out more about what might be preventing you from making the most of your experiences. Supposing, for example, you planned to spend an evening at the cinema with a friend, but then a colleague persuaded you to work late instead. Or supposing you planned to spend a whole morning catching up with a pile of post, but somehow you never got around to it.

In situations like these, where things do not work out as planned, you could ask yourself:

- What exactly was the problem?
- Did you overestimate what you could do in a particular chunk of time?
- Did you plan too much and exhaust yourself?
- Did you spend the day doing things you felt you *ought* to do, rather than things you would enjoy?
- Did you forget to include time for yourself or for relaxation?
- Or did you fritter away your time on nothing in particular and end up feeling you had had a wasted day?
- Did you end up doing what everyone else wanted, rather than what would have been good for you?

When you have identified the problem, ask yourself:

- Is this pattern familiar to you?
- Are there other situations in which you act in the same way?
- Could what went wrong with your plan reflect a more general Rule or strategy of yours (e.g. perfectionism or feeling you have to put others first)?

Once you understand the problem, you can begin to tackle it, by making practical changes and by identifying and re-thinking the self-defeating thoughts that are keeping you stuck. You may well find that what kept you from fulfilling your plan also gets in your way in other areas of your life.

What if I can't think of anything pleasurable to do?

It may be helpful to treat this difficulty as a special project: how many ways to enjoy yourself can you think of? Write down a list containing whatever comes to mind, however unlikely, without criticising or censoring it. You can work out the practicalities later. You can use the ideas below to help you, if you wish.

You could start by noticing what other people do for pleasure.

- What about your friends, and other people you know? What about what you see on television or social media?

_____

_____

_____

_____

_____

_____

- What about all the activities on the noticeboard in your local library, university or college of further education? And what about online? Does your town or neighbourhood have a 'What's On' website or app, for example?

_____

_____

_____

_____

_____

_____

- What do you notice people enjoying when you are out and about?

_____

_____

_____

_____

_____

_____

_____

Now turn your attention to yourself and add to your list.

- Even if you are not doing much for pleasure right now, have there been times in the past when you enjoyed certain activities? What were they?

_____

_____

_____

_____

_____

_____

_____

- Is there anything you have always fancied doing, but never got around to?

_____

_____

_____

_____

_____

- What are all the possible things you could do, even if you have never tried them?

_____

_____

_____

_____

_____

_____

Think of all the different pleasurable activities that might work for you under different circumstances.

- What could you do alone (e.g. reading, watching TV, going for walks)?

_____

_____

_____

_____

_____

_____

- What could you do with other people (e.g. going to the pub, joining an evening class, going to an art gallery)?

_____

_____

_____

_____

_____

_____

- What can you do that takes time (e.g. holidays, day trips, going to stay with people)?

_____

_____

_____

_____

_____

_____

- What can you do that can be easily fitted into the corners of your day (e.g. having a cup of special tea or a glass of special beer, soaking in a hot scented bath, pausing to glance out of the window)?

_____

_____

_____

_____

_____

_____

- What can you do that costs money (e.g. buying some flowers, going to the cinema, having a meal out)?

_____

_____

_____

_____

_____

_____

- What can you do that is free (e.g. looking at a sunset, window-shopping, looking through old photographs)?

_____

_____

_____

_____

_____

_____

- What physical pleasures can you think of (e.g. going swimming, flying a kite, having a massage)?

_____

_____

_____

_____

_____

_____

- What pleasures can you think of that use your mind (e.g. listening to a debate, doing a jigsaw or a crossword)?

_____

_____

_____

_____

_____

_____

- What can you do out of doors (e.g. taking care of your garden, going to the beach, going for a drive)?

_____

_____

_____

_____

_____

- And what can you do at home (e.g. choosing clothes from a catalogue, listening to music, playing computer games)?

_____

_____

_____

_____

Add all these things to your list.

Once you have a list of potential pleasures, plan them into your day. You may still have doubts about whether they will work for you. There is only one way to find out – experiments! And remember to watch out for killjoy thoughts. Put them to one side, if you can, and record and re-think them if they persist in getting in your way. When you give yourself pleasures like these, you are treating yourself like someone you love and care about. This is exactly the approach you need to take to enhance your self-esteem. It is OK to look after yourself, just as you would look after another person you loved and respected.

How can I deal with the fact that my day is genuinely full of obligations?

If your day is genuinely very busy with things you have to do, it can be difficult to make time for pleasure and relaxation. It may seem impossible even to fit in one more small thing. However, it is very important to realise that failing to make time just for yourself can backfire on you. If you keep draining water from a well, sooner or later it will run dry. You may find that you become increasingly tired and stressed so that, in the end, you are no longer able to do all the things you have to do as well as you would like to. Your health may even be affected. So finding time for relaxation is crucially important to your well-being and that of people around you.

If you accept that relaxation and pleasure are an essential part of caring for yourself, replenishing your resources and ensuring your health and well-being, you will be better able to make room for small pleasures, even on very busy days. Think of them as rewards for all your efforts, to which you are fully entitled. Take five minutes for a cup of coffee and a short walk. Take ten minutes for a shower with special soap. Choose something to eat for supper that you really like. Buy a small bunch of flowers that does not cost much. Listen to a favourite programme on the radio while you fix the car. Take advantage of your baby falling asleep to sit and read a magazine instead of feeling obliged to catch up with the housework. Be ingenious and creative, and don't allow yourself to be ground down by a relentless round of tasks and obligations. In the long run, you will not do yourself or anyone else any good.

How can I tackle all the things I have been putting off?

If you have been putting things off for a while, the prospect of facing them may seem rather daunting. However, tackling practical problems will enhance your sense of competence and so help to strengthen your self-esteem. By the same token, avoiding problems and tasks is likely to make you feel less in control of your life, and that will make you feel worse about yourself.

Follow these steps:

- Make a list of the tasks you have been putting off and problems you have been avoiding, in whatever order they occur to you.

- If you can, number the items on the list in order of importance. Which needs to be done first? And then what? And then what? If you cannot decide, or if it genuinely doesn't matter, simply put them in alphabetical order, or as they have occurred to you.

- Take the first task or problem on the list. Break it down into small, manageable steps. Rehearse the steps in your mind. As you do so, write down any practical problems you might encounter at each step and work out what to do about them. This may involve asking for help or advice or getting more information.

- As you rehearse what you plan to do, watch out for thoughts that make it difficult for you to problem-solve or tackle the task. You may find anxious predictions coming up (e.g. 'You won't be able to find a solution' or 'You'll never get everything done'). Or you may find yourself being self-critical (e.g. 'You should have dealt with this weeks ago' or 'You are a lazy slob'). If this happens, write your thoughts down and look for more helpful alternatives to them, as you have already learned to do.

- Once you have a step-by-step plan you feel reasonably

confident of, imagine following the steps through successfully as vividly as you can, just as an athlete imagines clearing the high jump or executing the perfect kick before actually doing it – and by doing so increases the chances of doing it success-fully in real life.

- Then tackle the task or problem one step at a time and deal with any practical difficulties and anxious or self-critical thoughts as they occur – just as you did in your rehearsal.

- Record the end result on your **Daily Activity Diary** and give yourself ratings for *Pleasure* and *Achievement*. Remember that even a small task completed, or a minor problem solved, deserves a pat on the back, if you have been putting it off!

- Take the next task on the list and tackle it in the same way.

Daily Activity Diary

	Monday	Tuesday	Wednesday	Thursday	Friday	Saturday	Sunday
6–7							
7–8							
8–9							
9–10							
10–11							
11–12							

MORNING

	12–1	1–2	2–3	3–4	4–5
A F T E R N O O N					

	Monday	Tuesday	Wednesday	Thursday	Friday	Saturday	Sunday
5–6							
6–7							
7–8							
8–9							
9–10							
10–11							

EVENING

11–12	
12–1	

Review: (What do you notice about your day? What worked for you? What did not work? What would you like to change?)

Mon:

Tues:

Weds:

Thurs:

Fri:

Sat:

Sun:

Daily Activity Diary

	Monday	Tuesday	Wednesday	Thursday	Friday	Saturday	Sunday
6–7							
7–8							
8–9							
9–10							
10–11							
11–12							

MORNING

	12–1	1–2	2–3	3–4	4–5
A F T E R N O O N					

	Monday	Tuesday	Wednesday	Thursday	Friday	Saturday	Sunday
5–6							
6–7							
7–8							
8–9							
9–10							
10–11							

EVENING

	11–12	12–1

Review: (What do you notice about your day? What worked for you? What did not work? What would you like to change?)

Mon:

Tues:

Weds:

Thurs:

Fri:

Sat:

Sun:

Daily Activity Diary

		Monday	Tuesday	Wednesday	Thursday	Friday	Saturday	Sunday
M O R N I N G	6–7							
	7–8							
	8–9							
	9–10							
	10–11							
	11–12							

12–1	1–2	2–3	3–4	4–5

A F T E R N O O N

		Monday	Tuesday	Wednesday	Thursday	Friday	Saturday	Sunday
EVENING	5–6							
	6–7							
	7–8							
	8–9							
	9–10							
	10–11							

11–12						
12–1						

Review: (What do you notice about your day? What worked for you? What did not work? What would you like to change?)

Mon:

Tues:

Weds:

Thurs:

Fri:

Sat:

Sun:

Daily Activity Diary

		Monday	Tuesday	Wednesday	Thursday	Friday	Saturday	Sunday
M O R N I N G	6–7							
	7–8							
	8–9							
	9–10							
	10–11							
	11–12							

12-1	1-2	2-3	3-4	4-5
A F T E R N O O N				

	Monday	Tuesday	Wednesday	Thursday	Friday	Saturday	Sunday
5–6							
6–7							
7–8							
8–9							
9–10							
10–11							

EVENING

| 11–12 | | | | | | | |
| 12–1 | | | | | | | |

Review: (What do you notice about your day? What worked for you? What did not work? What would you like to change?)

Mon:

Tues:

Weds:

Thurs:

Fri:

Sat:

Sun:

SUMMARY

1. Ignoring your good qualities, not allowing yourself to experience pleasure to the full, and discounting or denying your achievements, are part of the bias against yourself that keeps low self-esteem going.

2. To enhance your self-esteem, you need to learn to recognise and appreciate your good qualities and so develop a more balanced and kindly view of yourself. This complements the work you have already done to re-think self-critical thinking.

3. You can learn, step by step, to recognise, relive and record examples of your good points and positive qualities (the Good Points Chart). As you do so, accepting them (and so, accepting yourself) will become second nature.

4. You can also use a **Daily Activity Diary** to observe how you are spending your time and how much pleasure and sense of achievement you get from what you do. This gives you the information you need to start offering yourself a rich and satisfying life.

5. These changes are not always easy or straightforward. You can use the core skills you have already learned to tackle killjoy thoughts that get in your way.

6. The ultimate intention of this work is to learn to accept yourself for who you are and to feel worthy of treating yourself with the same kindness and consideration you would give to any other person you cared for.

THOUGHTS AND REFLECTIONS

THOUGHTS AND REFLECTIONS

PART THREE:

Changing the Rules, Creating a New Bottom Line, and Planning for the Future

Introduction

In Part One, we mapped out how low self-esteem develops and what keeps it going in the present day. In Part Two, we used this understanding to practise three core skills: awareness, re-thinking and experiments. The focus was on everyday patterns of thinking and behaviour which keep you stuck in low self-esteem – specifically, anxious predictions, self-critical thinking and difficulty in recognising your strengths and good qualities, and in treating yourself with the respect and kindness you would give to another person you cared about. Using the core skills gave you a chance to discover how to break the vicious circle of low self-esteem, to begin to learn to be your own good friend, treat yourself fairly, enjoy your life, and accept yourself just as you are.

But of course, as we saw in Part One, anxious predictions and self-critical thinking do not come out of the blue. They are the expression, in the present day, of central negative beliefs about yourself (the Bottom Line) and the Rules for Living you have developed in order to cope with them. In Part Three, it is time to begin to use the same core skills to tackle these broader ideas about yourself and how you must lead your life in order to feel OK about yourself. Finally, we shall look ahead and consider how best you can build on what you have learned as you worked your way through the handbook, and so continue your journey to healthy self-esteem.

SECTION 1:

Changing the Rules

In this section we shall begin work on an important barrier to self-acceptance: rigid, demanding Rules for Living. These may have been formed many years ago and are designed to help you get by in the world, given that your Bottom Line (your negative belief about yourself) appears to be true. In reality, they place heavy demands on you and restrict your life.

This section will help you to understand:

- where Rules for Living come from
- how to recognise Rules for Living
- how to identify your own Rules for Living
- how Rules for Living affect your daily life
- how to find new Rules for Living
- how to act on them

When you have low self-esteem, your Rules for Living determine the standards you expect of yourself, what you should do in order to be loved and accepted, and how you should behave in order to feel that you are a good and worthwhile person. These personal Rules demand that you 'keep to the straight and narrow' and give little room for manoeuvre or choice – this is how it *must* be. They often include a statement of what the consequences will be, if you fail to meet their terms. For instance, someone whose Bottom Line was 'I am unlovable' might have a Rule for Living that says: 'If I allow people to see my true self, they will reject me.'

Since the consequences of breaking such Rules are generally painful, you may have become very sensitive to situations where you are in danger of not meeting their terms. These are the situations that are likely to activate your Bottom Line, leading to the vicious circle of anxious predictions and self-critical thinking you were working on in Part Two. The flowchart that follows is a reminder of how this happens.

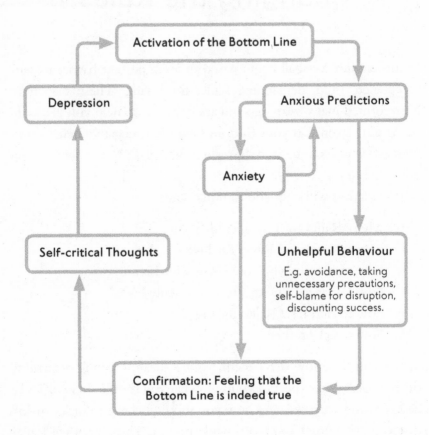

As you work through this section, it is worth summarising either on paper or electronically what you discover about each of your Rules, your line of argument when you question it, your new Rule, and your Action Plan for putting it into practice. You will find questions in this section, with spaces for you to write, and a summary worksheet on pp. 306–8 and also for download at www. overcoming.co.uk. These are designed to help you to organise your thoughts. This is important because unhelpful Rules for Living can be difficult to change – after all, you may have been putting them into practice, over and over again and in many different situations, for years. Recording your ideas as you go along will help you to keep your new perspective in view and make it easier for you to act on it, even when the going gets tough.

Where do Rules for Living come from?

Rules can be helpful. They enable us to make sense of what happens to us, to recognise repeating patterns, and to respond to new experiences without bewilderment. They can even help us to survive (e.g. 'I must always look both ways before crossing the road').

Parents pass on rules to their children, so that they will be able to deal with life independently (e.g. 'Make sure you eat a balanced diet'). Children also absorb rules from their families purely by observation. They notice connections (e.g. 'If I don't tidy my room, Mum will do it for me') and these can become a basis for more general rules (e.g. 'If things go wrong, someone will be there to pick up the pieces'). They notice what is praised and what is criticised, what brings a smile to a parent's face and what causes a frown. All these experiences can become a basis for personal Rules with a lasting impact on how people live their lives.

However, some Rules, instead of helping us to make sense of the world, trap us in unhelpful patterns and prevent us from achieving our life goals. They place demands on us that are impossible to meet and make no concessions to circumstances or individual needs (e.g. 'You must always give 110 per cent, no matter what the cost to yourself'). These extreme and unbending Rules create problems. They become a straitjacket, restricting freedom of movement and preventing change.

Rules that make you vulnerable to low self-esteem may determine the performance you expect of yourself in a range of different situations. Let's take Rajiv, from Part One, as an example. Here's a reminder of his story:

RAJIV'S STORY

Rajiv's father worked in a bank. He had never realised his ambitions to rise to a manager's position and put this down to the fact that his parents had failed to support him or show interest in what he was doing during his school years. So it was easy to skip school and neglect his homework. He was determined not to make the same mistake with his own children. Every supper time, he would question them about what they had learned. Everyone had to have an answer, and the answer had to be good enough.

Rajiv remembered dreading the daily grilling. He was sure his mind would go blank. When this happened, his father's face would fall in disappointment. Rajiv could see that he was letting his father down. 'If you can't do better than this,' his father would say, 'you'll never get anywhere in life.' In his heart of hearts, Rajiv agreed. It was clear to him that he was not good enough: he would never make it.

Rajiv's Bottom Line was 'I am not good enough' and his main Rule for Living was 'Unless I always get it right, I will never get anywhere in life'. This type of perfectionist Rule may not only require high-quality performance in the work environment, but might also require perfection in your physical appearance, in where you live or in how you carry out the most ordinary of everyday activities.

Rules can restrict your freedom to be your true self with other people. They may make you feel that approval, liking, love and intimacy are all dependent on your acting (or being) a certain way. Rules may even influence how you react to your own feelings and thoughts. For instance, you may base your good opinion of yourself on being fully in control of your emotions. But unhelpful Rules like these imprison you. They build a wall of expectations and demands around you. This is your chance to break out.

Rules for Living and the Bottom Line

At the heart of low self-esteem is your belief that your Bottom Line is true. Rules for Living are like 'escape clauses', ways to get round the Bottom Line. For example, at heart, you might believe yourself to be incompetent. But *so long as* you work very hard all the time and set yourself high standards, you can override your incompetence and feel OK about yourself. Or you might believe yourself to be unattractive. But *so long as* you are the life and soul of the party, maybe no one will notice and once again you can feel OK about yourself.

Rules like these can work very well, much of the time – which is why we carry on obeying them. For long periods, they may protect you from the pain of low self-esteem. But there is a fundamental problem. Such Rules allow you to wallpaper over what you feel to be the real truth about yourself (your Bottom Line). But they do not change it. Indeed, the more successful they are, and the better you are at meeting their demands, the less opportunity they give you to stand back, question your Bottom Line, and accept yourself as you are. So, the Bottom Line stays there, waiting to be wheeled into place whenever your Rules are in danger of being broken. On p. 265 you can see how this worked for Rajiv.

How can you recognise Rules for Living?

Rules are learned

Unhelpful personal Rules are rarely formally taught but tend to be absorbed through experience and observation. This is rather like a child learning to speak without learning the formal rules of grammar.

Personal Rules for Living are often the same – you may consistently act in accordance with them, without having ever expressed them in so many words. This is probably because they reflect decisions you made about how to operate in the world, when you were very young. Your Rules probably made perfect sense when you drew them up, but they were based on the limited experience available to you at the time, and so may be out of date and irrelevant to your life now.

Rules are part of the culture we grow up in

Our social and family heritage is comprised of rules. For example, society has evolved certain rules about how men and women should act. We absorb these ideas from our earliest years and, even if we disagree with them, it may be difficult to act against them. We may be punished for attempting to do so by social disapproval. The difficulties women still have in reaching senior positions in the workplace, and the struggle to establish a meaningful role for men in childcare, would be examples of this.

Personal Rules are often like exaggerated versions of the rules of the society we grew up in. Western society, for example, places a high value on independence and achievement. In a particular individual, these social pressures might be expressed through Rules like 'I must never ask for help' or 'If I'm not on top, I'm a flop'. However, social and cultural rules can change, and such changes (via the family) will have an impact on personal Rules. The English, for example, used to be famous for their 'stiff upper lip' stoicism. In the individual, this might be expressed as: 'If I show my feelings, people will write me off as a wimp.' More recently, however, things have changed and the value of openly expressing vulnerability and emotion has come to the fore. In the individual, this might become: 'If I do not lay all my feelings on the table, it means I am hard and inhuman.' Whatever your background, the chances are that your personal Rules reflect the culture you grew up in, as well as that of your immediate family.

Rajiv's Rules for Living and his Bottom Line

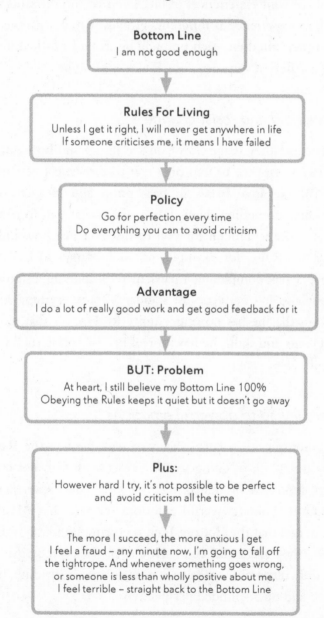

Your Rules are unique to you

Although your Rules may have much in common with those of other people growing up in the same culture, no one else will exactly share your experiences of life. Even within the same family, each child's experience is different. However much parents try to be fair to their children, each one will be treated a little differently, loved in a different way. So, your Rules are unique.

Rules are rigid and resist change

This is because they shape how you see things and how you make sense of what happens to you on a day-to-day basis (see Part One, Section 3). Negative biases in perception and in interpretation reinforce and strengthen them. Rules encourage you to behave in ways that make it difficult for you to discover just how unhelpful they are. So, Rajiv, for example, not only strives to be '100 per cent great' when completing a particularly important assignment at work, but also has perfectionist standards for everything he does. This means that he has no opportunity to discover that, given his natural talents and skills, he has no real need to place such pressure on himself.

Rules are linked to powerful emotions

Strong emotions are a signal that you have broken the Rules, or that you are at risk of doing so. You react with fear, not concern. You feel depressed or despairing, not sad. You experience rage, not irritation. These powerful emotions tell you that a Rule is in operation, and that the Bottom Line is gearing up for activation. In this sense, they are useful clues. However, their strength may also make it difficult to observe what is going on with curiosity, from an interested and open-minded perspective.

Rules are unreasonable

Like anxious predictions and self-critical thoughts, personal Rules for Living do not match the facts. They do not fit the way the world works, or what can reasonably be expected of any normal, imperfect human being. Rajiv (p. 265) recognises this point when he acknowledges that it is not always possible to be perfect or to avoid criticism. We shall return to this point in more detail when we come to reformulate your personal Rules.

Rules are extreme

Unhelpful Rules are over-generalisations. They do not recognise that what is helpful changes according to the circumstances in which you find yourself. They do not respond to variations in time and place or recognise that what works at one time of your life will not work at another. This is reflected in their language: 'always'/'never', 'everyone'/'no one', 'everything'/'nothing'. They prevent you from selecting the best course of action, flexibly responding according to your particular needs at a particular moment in time.

Rules are absolute; they do not allow for shades of grey. This too is reflected in their language: 'I must . . . ', 'I should . . . ', 'I ought to . . . ', rather than 'I would like to . . . ', I want . . . ', 'I prefer . . . ', 'It would be in my best interests to . . . '. This may be because they were developed when you were very young, before you had the breadth of experience to see things from a more complex perspective.

Rules are based on things that cannot be guaranteed

The sequence Rajiv identified on p. 265 illustrates an important point. He noticed that his Rules required something that was in fact impossible: unfailing 100 per cent performance and never encountering criticism of any kind. This is characteristic of unhelpful Rules linked to low self-esteem. They mean that your sense of your own worth is dependent on things that are impossible (e.g. being perfect, always being in full control of what happens to you), or outside your control (e.g. being accepted and liked by everyone).

People hang self-esteem on a whole range of pegs:

• Being young • Being beautiful • Being fit and healthy • Being in paid employment • Being a parent • Having money • Having social status • Being at the right school or college • Having a partner	• Being a particular weight or shape • Being top dog • Achieving success • Being famous • Being loved • Having children who are doing well • Being secure • Being sexually attractive, and so on

The list is endless. But none of these things can be guaranteed. We all get old; we all get sick from time to time; we may be damaged or disabled; we may lose our employment (whether through company relocation, economic downturn or even planned retirement); our children leave home (or if they don't, that becomes a cause of concern); there are times in our lives when we have no one special to love us or when our futures are insecure; and so on. All these things are fragile and could be taken away. This means that, if we depend on them in order to feel good about ourselves, our self-esteem is also fragile. To be happy with yourself simply for existing, just as you are, regardless of your circumstances, puts you in a far stronger position.

How to identify your Rules for Living (Awareness)

You are looking for general Rules that reflect what you expect of yourself, your standards for how you should behave, your sense of what is acceptable and what is not allowed, and your idea of what is necessary in order to succeed in life and achieve satisfying relationships. In essence, you are defining what you have to do or be in order to feel good about yourself. If you have low self-esteem, the chances are that these standards are demanding and unrealistic (more, for example, than you would expect of any other person) and that, when you explore their impact, you will discover that they actually prevent you from having a secure sense that it is OK to be you.

Rules for Living are usually expressed in one of three ways: assumptions, drivers and value judgements.

Assumptions

These are your ideas about the connections between self-esteem and other things in life. These usually take the form of 'If . . . , then . . . ' statements. (They can also be phrased as 'Unless . . . , then . . . '.)

Here are some examples of assumptions:

- *If* I allow anyone to get close to me, *[then]* they will hurt and exploit me (Briony)
- *If* someone criticises me, *[then]* it means I have failed (Rajiv)
- *Unless* I do everything people expect of me, *[then]* I will be rejected (Kate)
- Nothing I do is worthwhile *unless* it is recognised by others (i.e. *Unless* what I do is recognised by others, *[then]* it is not worthwhile) (Lin)

Assumptions like these are rather like anxious predictions. They describe what you think will happen if you act (or fail to act) in a certain way. This immediately provides a clue to one important way of changing them: experiments. They can be tested by setting up the

'If . . . ' and seeing if the 'then . . . ' really happens. As we learned with anxious predictions, the threat could be more apparent than real.

Drivers

These are the 'shoulds', 'musts' and 'oughts' that compel us to act in particular ways, or be particular kinds of people, in order to feel good about ourselves. Drivers usually link up with a hidden *'or else . . .'*. Here are some examples:

- I must never let anyone see my true self (*or else they will see what a bad person I am and reject me*) (Briony)
- I must always keep myself under tight control (*or else I will go over the top and spoil things*) (Jack)
- I should be able to cope with anything life throws at me (*or else I am pathetic*) (Mike)

You can see from these examples that the *'or else . . . '* may be very close to the Bottom Line. In fact, the *'or else . . . '* may be a simple statement of the Bottom Line: *'or else . . . it means that I am inadequate/unlovable/incompetent/ugly'* or whatever.

Value judgements

These are statements about how it would be if you acted (or did not act) in a particular way, or if you were (or were not) a particular kind of person. In a sense, these are rather similar to assumptions, but their terms are less clear, and may need to be questioned in order to be fully understood. Examples would be: 'It's terrible to make mistakes', 'Being rejected is unbearable', 'It's vital to be on top of things'. If you find Rules that take this form, you need to ask yourself some questions in order to find out what exactly you mean by these vague words ('terrible', 'unbearable', 'vital'). For example:

- What's 'terrible' about mistakes? If I did make one, what then?

What would it say about me? What is the worst that could happen? What would the consequences be?

- What do I mean by 'unbearable'? If I imagine being rejected, what exactly comes to mind? What do I see happening? How do I think I would feel? And for how long?
- 'Vital' in what way? What would happen if I were not on top of things? What does being on top protect me from? What is the worst that could happen if I was not? What sort of person would it make me? What impact would it have on my place in the world?

How will you know when you have found your Rules?

Discovering your Rules is a fascinating process. You become like a detective, searching for clues. Once again, see if you can go about this with a sense of interest and curiosity. Just what is going on here? What exactly are your repeating patterns? What do they tell you about what you must do or be in order to feel OK about yourself?

You may even be quite surprised to discover what your Rules are ('Oh, that's nonsense, I don't believe that'). If this is your first reaction, stop for a moment and consider. It may be hard to believe your Rule when you are sitting calmly with it written down in front of you. But what about when you are in a situation relevant to it? For example, if your Rule is to do with pleasing people, what about situations where you feel you have not done so? Or if your Rule is to do with success, what about situations where you feel you have failed? Even if the Rule you have identified does not seem fully convincing to you in the cold light of day, do you in fact *act and feel as if it were true?* If so, then – unlikely as it may seem – you've struck gold.

When it comes to identifying your Rules, you already have a wealth of relevant information from the work you have done on anxious predictions, self-critical thoughts and enhancing self-acceptance. You may already have observed that certain situations always spark off uncomfortable emotions and cause you problems. These are likely to be the situations relevant to your own personal set of Rules. Key situations for Rajiv, for example, were times when he might be unable to perform to a high standard and feared he would attract criticism.

Your observation of repeating patterns in your reactions may have already given you a pretty clear idea of what your Rules are. If not, don't worry. If you have never put them into words, it may take a while to find the right phrasing. Be creative and open-minded. Approach the task from different angles, using the ideas below to develop hunches as to what they might be. Try different Rules on for size, experiment with different wordings, and use all the clues at your disposal, until you find a general statement which seems to have been influencing you more or less consistently for some time, and which has affected your life in many different situations.

Although you may have a number of Rules, it is probably best to work systematically on one at a time. Choose a Rule that relates to an area of your life that you particularly want to change (e.g. relationships with other people). When you have completed the process of formulating an alternative Rule and trying it out in practice, you can use what you have learned to tackle other unhelpful Rules that you also wish to change.

SOURCES OF INFORMATION

You can use a number of sources of information to identify your Rules:

1. Direct statements
2. Themes
3. Your judgements of yourself and other people
4. Memories, family sayings
5. Follow the opposite (things you feel really good about)
6. Downward arrow

---

1 Direct statements

- Look through the record you kept of your anxious predictions and self-critical thoughts in Part Two of the book and see if you can identify any Rules disguised as specific thoughts.
- Do any of your predictions in particular situations reflect broader issues?
- Are any of your self-critical thoughts specific examples of a more general Rule?

_____

_____

_____

_____

_____

_____

2 Themes

- Even if no Rules for Living are directly stated in your record sheets, can you pick out continuing preoccupations and concerns? Or repeating themes that run through the work you have done?
- What kinds of situations always make you doubt yourself (e.g. noticing you have not done something well, or having to encounter people you are unfamiliar with)?
- What aspects of yourself are you most hard on?
- What behaviour in other people undermines your confidence?

_____

_____

_____

_____

_____

_____

3 Your judgements of yourself and other people

- Look at your self-critical thoughts and ask yourself under what circumstances you begin to put yourself down?
- What do you criticise in yourself?
- What does that tell you about what you expect of yourself?
- What might happen if you relaxed your standards?
- How could things go wrong?
- If you do not keep a tight rein on yourself and obey the Rule, where will you end up? What sort of person might you become (e.g. stupid, lazy, selfish)?
- What are you never allowed to do or be, no matter what?
- What standards do you expect other people to meet? (These may reflect the demands you place on yourself.)

_____

_____

_____

_____

_____

_____

_____

_____

_____

4 Memories, family sayings

Think back to when you were young, as a child and in your teens, and consider the messages you received about how to behave and the sort of person you should be. When you were growing up:

- What were you told you should and should not do?
- What were the consequences if you did not go along with what you were told? What sort of person did that make you? What were you told to expect? What were the implications for your relationships with other people, or for your future?
- What were you criticised or punished or ridiculed for?
- What did people say or do when you did not make the grade, or failed to meet expectations?
- How did people who were important to you react when you made mistakes, or were naughty, or did not do well at school?
- What were you praised and appreciated for?
- What did you have to do or be in order to receive warmth and affection?
- What family proverbs and sayings can you remember (e.g. 'Better safe than sorry', 'I want doesn't get', 'Stupid is as stupid does')?

_____

_____

_____

_____

_____

_____

_____

_____

_____

To help you search out memories of particular experiences, look at your thought records again, and pick out feelings and thoughts that seem typical to you (themes). Ask yourself:

- When did you first have those feelings, or notice yourself thinking and behaving in that way? What were the circumstances?
- When you look at something that usually makes you anxious or triggers self-criticism, does this remind you of anything in your past? Whose voices or faces come to mind?
- When did you first grasp that certain things were expected of you, or get the sense that approval or love depended on something you were required to do or be, rather than simply on the fact that you existed?
- What particular memories or images or sayings come to mind?

5 Follow the opposite

Think about the times when you have felt particularly good, and ask yourself:

- What makes you feel really, really good?
- What are the implications of this? What Rule might you have obeyed? What standards did you meet?
- What qualities and actions do you really admire and value in other people? What does this tell you about how *you* are supposed to act or be?

_____

_____

_____

_____

_____

_____

_____

6 Downward Arrow

This is a way of using your awareness of how you think and feel in specific problem situations to get at general Rules. Here is Rajiv's Downward Arrow, as an example:

Situation:
Was asked a question I could not answer in a meeting

Emotions:
Anxious, self-conscious, embarrassed

Body Sensations:
Hot, tight jaw and hands

Thought:
'I should know the answer to that'

↓

What does it mean to me that I don't?

↓

'That I'm not doing my job properly'

↓

And if that was true, what would it mean to me?

↓

'That sooner or later people will notice that I'm not up to it'

↓

And supposing they did, what would follow on from that?

↓

'I would lose credibility. I might be demoted'

↓

And what are the implications of all that for my performance?

↓

'I really can't afford not to have the answers to everything.
I've got to come up with the goods, all the time, no matter what'

↓

So what's the Rule?
Unless I always get it right, I will never get anywhere in life

You will find **Downward Arrow Charts** to fill in on pp. 279–81. There is an extra one at the back of the book which you can photocopy if you wish, and it is also available for download at www.overcoming.co.uk.

RULES FOR LIVING DOWNWARD ARROW CHART

Situation:_____

Emotions: _____

Key thought:_____

What does this mean to you?

↓

_____

_____

↓

And if that was true, what would it mean to you?

↓

_____

_____

↓

And supposing that happened, what would it mean to you?

↓

_____

_____

↓

And what would that mean to you?

↓

_____

_____

↓

So, what's the Rule?

↓

_____

_____

RULES FOR LIVING DOWNWARD ARROW CHART

Situation:_____

Emotions:_____

Key thought:_____

What does this mean to you?

↓

_____

_____

↓

And if that was true, what would it mean to you?

↓

_____

_____

↓

And supposing that happened, what would it mean to you?

↓

_____

_____

↓

And what would that mean to you?

↓

_____

_____

↓

So, what's the Rule?

↓

_____

_____

RULES FOR LIVING DOWNWARD ARROW CHART

Situation:_____

Emotions: _____

Key thought:_____

What does this mean to you?

↓

_____

_____

↓

And if that was true, what would it mean to you?

↓

_____

_____

↓

And supposing that happened, what would it mean to you?

↓

_____

_____

↓

And what would that mean to you?

↓

_____

_____

↓

So, what's the Rule?

↓

_____

_____

Some guidelines for using the Downward Arrow Charts:

How many steps?

Rajiv reached his Rule in five steps – but you may find it takes you more or fewer than that. Don't feel that you should have got there by a certain number of steps. Sometimes Rules come into focus very quickly, but other times not, especially if you have never really put them into words.

Starting point: Trigger situations

Start by thinking of the kind of problem situation that always upsets you and makes you feel bad about yourself (e.g. being criticised, failing to meet a deadline, avoiding an opportunity). These are the situations where your Bottom Line has been activated because you are in danger of breaking your Rules or have actually broken them.

Now think of a recent example that is still fresh in your memory. Call the example vividly to mind, as if you were experiencing it over again. What exactly was the situation? What thoughts or images were running through your mind? What emotions did you experience? And what body sensations? And what was the outcome? Write down what you remember, in detail. When you have done so, identify the thought or image that seems to you to be most important, and that most fully accounts for how you felt and what you did.

Then, rather than starting to re-think the key thought, ask yourself: 'Supposing that thought or image were true, what would it mean to me?' When you find your answer to this question, ask the question again: 'And supposing that were true, what would it mean to me?' Continue on, step by step, until you discover the general underlying Rule that makes sense of your thoughts and feelings in the specific problem situation you started from. Remember, you are looking for assumptions ('If..., then . . . '), drivers ('I should . . . ', 'I must . . . ', 'I ought . . . ') or value judgements ('It's great/terrible if . . . ').

Helpful questions

'What would that mean to you?' is just one possible question you can use to pursue the downward arrow. Here are some others that may be helpful:

- Supposing that were true, what would it mean to you?
- Supposing that were true, what would happen then? What would follow from that?
- What are the implications of that?
- What's the worst that might happen? And what would happen then? And then?
- What would be so bad about that? (NB: 'I would feel bad' is not a helpful answer to this question. You probably would feel bad, but that does not tell you anything useful or interesting about your Rules. So, if your immediate answer is something about your own feelings, ask yourself *why* you would feel bad.)
- How would that be a problem for you?
- What does that tell you about how you should behave?
- What does that tell you about what you expect from yourself, or from other people?
- What does that tell you about your standards for yourself?
- What does that tell you about the sort of person you should be in order to feel good about yourself?
- What does that tell you about what you must do or be, in order to gain the acceptance, approval, liking or love of other people?
- What does that tell you about what you must do or be in order to succeed in life?

Recognising when you have reached the Rule

If, when you do the downward arrow, you have a sense of going round in circles after a certain point, the chances are that you have reached your Rule, but that it is not in a form you can easily recognise. In this case, stop questioning, stand back and reflect on your sequence. What Rule for Living do the final levels suggest to you? When you have an idea, try the draft Rule on for size. Can you think of other situations where this might apply? Does it make sense of how you operate elsewhere?

Try another similar starting point. Does it end up in the same place? Take a few days to observe yourself, especially your anxious predictions and self-critical thoughts. Does your draft Rule make sense of your everyday reactions? If so, you are in a position to start looking for a more helpful alternative. If not, what Rule might better account for what you observe? Don't be discouraged; have another go.

You may find at first that you have a good general sense of what your Rule might be, but that the way you have expressed it doesn't feel quite right. If so, play around with the wording until you find a version that 'clicks' with you. Try out the different possible forms a Rule can take: assumptions, drivers and value judgements. When you get the right wording, you will experience a sense of recognition – 'Aha! So that's what it is.'

Remember, you may well have a number of unhelpful Rules for Living – people often do. In this case, you might find it interesting to pursue downward arrows from several different starting points. This is crucial if you have difficulty identifying your Rule when you first do it. It is also a way of checking that you are on the right track, and of discovering your other Rules. Experiment with asking different questions, too. The answers may be illuminating.

How do Rules for Living affect your everyday life?

Rules may influence how you think, feel and act in a whole range of different situations, and over time. As we said, you may well have learned them when you were very young.

Once you have identified an unhelpful Rule, it is worth considering the impact it has had on your life. When you come to change your Rule, you will not only need to formulate a more realistic and helpful alternative, but also to modify its continued influence on your daily life. Recognising the old Rule's impact will help you to achieve this. You will already have much of the information you need, from the work you have done on anxious predictions, self-critical thoughts and enhancing self-esteem.

Start by looking at your life now. Ask yourself:

How does your Rule affect your relationships?

_____

_____

_____

_____

_____

_____

_____

_____

How does it affect your study or your work?

_____

_____

_____

_____

_____

_____

_____

How does it affect how you spend your leisure time?

_____

_____

_____

_____

_____

How does it affect how well you look after yourself?

_____

_____

_____

_____

_____

_____

_____

How does it affect how you react when things don't go well?

_____

_____

_____

_____

_____

How does it affect how you respond to opportunities and challenges?

_____

_____

_____

_____

_____

_____

_____

How does it affect how good you are at expressing your feelings and making sure your needs are met?

_____

_____

_____

_____

_____

_____

_____

How do you know your Rule is in operation? What are the clues?

_____

_____

_____

_____

_____

_____

What emotions do you experience?

_____

_____

_____

_____

_____

_____

_____

What sensations do you notice in your body?

_____

_____

_____

_____

_____

_____

_____

What usually runs through your mind (thoughts, images)?

_____

_____

_____

_____

_____

_____

_____

What do you do (or fail to do)?

_____

_____

_____

_____

_____

_____

_____

What reactions do you get from other people?

_____

_____

_____

_____

_____

_____

_____

Now look back over time. Can you see a similar pattern extending into your past? What effect has the Rule had on you, over the course of your life?

What unnecessary precautions has it led you to take?

_____

_____

_____

_____

_____

_____

What have you missed out on, or failed to take advantage of, or lost because of the Rule?

_____

_____

_____

_____

_____

_____

What restrictions has it placed on you?

_____

_____

_____

_____

_____

_____

How has it stopped you appreciating yourself and relaxing with others?

_____

_____

_____

_____

_____

How has it affected your ability to experience pleasure?

_____

_____

_____

_____

_____

Look back at the work you have already done on anxious predictions, self-critical thinking and self-acceptance. How much of what
you have observed can be accounted for by this Rule?

_____

_____

_____

_____

_____

_____

_____

After this detailed investigation, you should now have a good sense of what your Rule (or Rules) might be. Use the first three headings on the worksheet on p. 306 to summarise in writing what you have discovered:

1. My old Rule is (state it in your own words):
2. This Rule has had the following impact on my life (summarise the ways in which it has affected you):
3. I know the Rule is in operation, because (note the clues that tell you your Rule is active – feelings, sensations, thoughts, patterns of behaviour):

Changing the Rules: Re-thinking and experiments

Now that you know what your Rules are, it's time to change them and seek new ones that are more realistic and constructive. You can use the same core skills that you practised when you tackled anxious predictions and self-critical thoughts, and when you learned to acknowledge your good points and treat yourself with respect and kindness. Here are some questions that may be helpful:

- Where did the Rule come from?
- In what ways is it unreasonable?
- What are the advantages of obeying it?
- What are the disadvantages of obeying it?
- How can you chart its advantages and disadvantages?
- What alternative Rule would be more realistic and helpful?
- What do you need to do to 'test drive' your new Rule? How can you go about putting it into practice on a day-to-day basis?

Your aim is to find new Rules that will encourage you to adopt more realistic and compassionate standards for yourself and help you to get what you want out of life. As we said earlier, you may have discovered more than one unhelpful Rule that keeps your self-esteem low (for example, perhaps you need approval and you are also something of a perfectionist). If so, start with the one you would most like to change, and then use what you learn to undermine the others. You will gain more from working systematically on one Rule at a time than from jumping around from one to another, doing a little bit here and a little bit there.

Use the spaces provided below to note down your ideas in detail. Then, just as you did with your investigations earlier on, summarise your thoughts on the worksheet on pp. 306.

1 Where did the Rule come from?

The purpose here is not to wallow in the past, but to understand how your Rules started and what has kept them going. This will help you to step back from them and see them simply as out-of-date strategies which you no longer need to obey. Keep these questions in mind:

- How far does my past experience explain my Rules?
- How well does it explain the strategies I have adopted?
- How well does it help me to understand how I operate now?

Understanding the origins of your Rules will help you to see that they were your best options, given the knowledge available to you at the time. This insight can be a helpful first step towards updating them. However, if you cannot think where they have come from, do not despair. This information is not essential to changing them. It just means that the questions that follow are likely to be more helpful to you.

If you can, summarise for yourself the experiences in your life that led to the Rule. Remind yourself when you first noticed the signs that tell you it is in operation.

- Was the Rule part of your family culture, or part of the wider culture in which you grew up?
- Did you adopt it as a means of dealing with difficult and distressing circumstances?
- Was it a way of gaining the closeness and caring you needed as a child?
- Or was it a way of managing unkind or unpredictable adults?
- Or coping with the demands of school?
- Or avoiding teasing and ridicule?

_____

_____

_____

_____

_____

_____

You may also want to take into account later experiences that have helped to keep the Rule in place.

- For example, have you found yourself trapped in abusive relationships?
- Have other people taken over the critical role your parents took towards you?
- Have you repeatedly found yourself in situations that reinforce the policies you have adopted?

_____

_____

_____

_____

_____

_____

_____

Even though the Rule did make sense at one point, you neverthe-less need to ask yourself how relevant it is to you now, as an adult.

- Is it still necessary or beneficial?
- Or might you in fact be better off with an updated perspective?

_____

_____

_____

_____

_____

_____

2 In what ways is the Rule unreasonable?

Call on your adult knowledge and life experience to consider in what ways your Rule fails to take account of how the world works.

- How does it go beyond what is realistically possible for an ordin-ary, imperfect human being?
- How does it go beyond what you would expect from another person you respected and cared about?
- In what ways are its demands over the top, exaggerated or im-possible to meet?

_____

_____

_____

_____

_____

_____

_____

Remember, this was a contract you made with yourself as a child.

- Would you now allow a child to run your life for you?
- Why not?
- What can you see as an adult that you could not grasp when you were very young?

_____

_____

_____

_____

_____

_____

3 What are the advantages of obeying the Rule?

It is important to be clear about the benefits of following your present Rules, because the alternatives you formulate will need to give you the payoffs of the old Rule, without its disadvantages. Otherwise, you may be understandably reluctant to change.

Make a list of the advantages of your present Rule.

- What benefits do you gain from it?
- In what ways is it helpful to you?
- What might you risk if you were to let go of it?
- What does it protect you from?

_____

_____

_____

_____

_____

_____

_____

People often worry that if they were to abandon their Rules, catastrophe would follow. For instance, Rajiv's high standards genuinely motivated him to do excellent work, for which he was respected and praised, and which has helped to advance his career. So, letting go of them felt like a major risk. He suspected that if he were not a perfectionist, he might never again do a decent piece of work. And it felt to him as though his perfectionism was the only thing that guaranteed acceptance from other people. Ideas like these can be tested out through experiments at a later stage. For the moment, the important thing is to identify the advantages and fears that keep the old Rule in place.

When you have listed all the advantages of your Rule, take a careful look at them. Some of them may be more apparent than real. For example, the Rule that you must always put others first may encourage you to be genuinely helpful and dispose others to feel kindly towards you. But there may be a downside: your own needs are not met, and you may end up feeling increasingly resentful and exhausted, so that in the end you are no longer in a fit state to look after others. Rajiv realised, on reflection, that his excellent work did not in fact always guarantee acceptance. He was sometimes so driven and tense that people found him unapproachable and thought him arrogant.

Do not take the advantages you have identified for granted. Look at them closely and assess how genuine they are. Do the same for your concerns about dropping your Rule.

- How do you know these things would actually happen?
- How could you find out?

_____

_____

_____

_____

_____

_____

_____

_____

4 What are the disadvantages of obeying the Rule?

You have explored the apparent payoffs; now for the downside. Examine the ways in which the Rule robs you of pleasure, sours your relationships with other people, undermines your sense of achievement or stands in the way of getting what you want out of life. Use the information you collected when you were assessing its impact on your life (see pp. 284–291).

_____

_____

_____

_____

_____

_____

_____

Make a list of some of your main goals in life (e.g. to have a satisfying career; to take pleasure in what you do; to be relaxed and confident with people; to make the most of every experience). Then ask yourself:

- Does this Rule help me to reach these goals?
- Is it the best strategy for getting what I most value in life?
- Or does it in fact stand in my way?

_____

_____

_____

_____

_____

_____

_____

_____

_____

5 How to chart the advantages and disadvantages

Use the chart on the next page. Summarise the advantages and disadvantages you have identified by writing the apparent advantages attached to your Rule and the apparent risks of letting it go, in the left-hand column. Then list its disadvantages, in the right-hand column.

Now weigh up the two lists and write your conclusions about how helpful your Rule actually is underneath. If you decide that, on balance, it *is* helpful, then you need take this exercise no further. If, on the other hand, you conclude that it is *un*helpful, and stands in the way of getting what you want out of life, you need to formulate an alternative that will give you the advantages of the old Rule without its disadvantages.

Advantages of the Rule	Disadvantages of the Rule

Conclusions

6 What alternative Rule would be more realistic and helpful?

New Rules can transform day-to-day experiences. They allow you to deal comfortably and confidently with situations that, under the old system, would have triggered anxiety or self-criticism. What would have been disasters become passing inconveniences. What would have seemed matters of life and death become exciting challenges and opportunities. In essence, you are seeking a new Rule that will allow you more freedom of movement to be yourself, a Rule that encourages you to accept and appreciate yourself just as you are.

IT'S WORTH REMEMBERING . . .

New Rules can open the door to accepting yourself and attaining what is most important to you in life.

To help you to free up your thinking, consider whether you would advise another person to adopt your old Rule as a policy. Would you want to pass it on to a good friend, or to your children, if you had any? If not, what would you prefer their Rule to be?

Your new Rule will probably be more flexible and realistic than the old one, better able to take account of variations in circumstances, and to operate in terms of 'some of the people, some of the time' rather than 'everyone, always'. It will inhabit the middle ground rather than the extremes. So, it may begin:

- 'I want to . . . '
- 'I enjoy . . . '
- 'I prefer . . . '
- 'It's OK to . . . '

rather than:

- 'I must . . . '

- 'I should . . . '
- 'I ought to . . . '
- 'It would be terrible if . . . '

You may find that your new Rule starts with the same 'If . . . ', but ends with a different 'then . . . '. For example, Rajiv replaced 'If someone criticises me, it means I have failed' with 'If someone criticises me, I may or may not deserve it. If I have done something worthy of criticism, that's not failure – it's all part of being human, and an opportunity to learn, and there's nothing wrong with that.'

This example illustrates something typical of new Rules: they are often longer and more elaborate than old ones. This is because they are based on an adult's ability to understand how the world works, and to take into account variations in circumstances. Sometimes it is nice, however, to capture their essence in a slogan, the sort of snappy statement you might find on a badge or T-shirt. Sometime after he had formulated his new Rule, Rajiv watched a film in which a young boy was struggling to please his father on the mistaken grounds that only something exceptional would win his approval. Rajiv decided to adopt the father's loving response as a slogan for himself: 'You don't have to be great, to be great.'

You may find it difficult at first to find an alternative you feel comfortable with. Once you have what feels like a reasonably good draft, it can be very helpful to use your imagination to get a feel for how it might work in practice (a sort of virtual experiment). Go back to the problematic situation that was the starting point for your Downward Arrow. Supposing your new Rule had been in place at that time, how would it have changed things? Imagine as vividly as you can what sort of thoughts, feelings and body sensations might have been present, and how you might have acted differently. Would things have played out differently and better if you had been operating from your new Rule? If yes, then it's time to experiment for real. If no, then time to have a re-think.

Once you have something that feels workable, write it down and then try putting it into operation for a week or two to find out how well it works for you in real situations and if there are any ways of changing it for the better. It may also be worth talking to and observing other people. What do you think their Rules might be? Your observations will give you an opportunity to discover the different positions people adopt, and to clarify what strategy might work best for you.

How to put your new Rules for Living into practice (Experiments)

Your old Rule may have been in operation for a long time. In contrast, the new one is freshly made, and it may take a while for it to become a comfortable fit. What can you do to consolidate your new policy, check out how well it works for you, and start putting it into practice in your everyday life? This takes us back to all the work you have already done, and to the central idea of finding things out for yourself by setting up experiments and examining their outcomes. The most important thing you can do to strengthen your new Rule (and indeed to discover if you need to make further changes to it) is to act as if it was true and observe the outcome. This is where we shall go next. But first, it is worth consolidating what you have already discovered so that you have a sound basis for creating effective experiments.

Consolidating what you have learned

The written summary

This is a good time to complete your written summary, using the headings on the worksheet on pp. 306–8 if you wish, and either on paper or electronically. The summary will give you a concise version of the work you have done on your Rule, all in one place. This will make it easy for you to review and refer to it as you continue to work on finding more flexible and helpful strategies. (You will find a copy of Rajiv's written summary on pp. 319–322, just before the Section Summary.)

You have already summarised your findings in relation to recognising the Rule and its impact on your life. Now continue with the work you have done on investigating where it came from, its shortcomings, and your new Rule:

1. It is understandable that I have this Rule because (summarise the experiences that led to the development of the Rule and that have reinforced it):

2. However, the Rule is unreasonable because (summarise the ways in which your Rule does not fit the way the world works):

3. The advantages of obeying the Rule are (summarise the advantages of obeying the Rule and the risks of letting it go. Check to see if these are genuine):

4. But the disadvantages are (summarise the harmful effects of obeying the Rule):

5. A more realistic and helpful Rule would be (write out your new Rule, in your own words):

6. In order to test-drive the new Rule, I need to (write down how you plan to strengthen your new Rule and act on it in everyday life):

Like your list of positive qualities and good points, a written summary on its own is not enough. Your new Rule needs to be part of your everyday awareness, so that it has the best possible chance of influencing your feelings and thoughts and what you do in problem situations. So, when you have completed your summary, put it somewhere easily accessible and, over the next few weeks, read it carefully every day, letting it sink in – perhaps more than once a day, to begin with. A good time is just after you get up. This puts you in the right frame of mind for the day. Another good time is just before you go to bed, when you can think over your day and consider how the work you have done is changing things for you.

The objective is to make your new Rule part of your mental furniture so that acting in accordance with it eventually becomes second nature. Continue to read your summary regularly until you find you have reached this point.

The flashcard

Another helpful way to encourage the changes you are trying to make is to write your new Rule on a stiff or laminated card that is small enough to be easily carried in a wallet or purse. Or you could have it as wallpaper on your computer or program it to pop up at intervals on your smartphone. You can use these prompts to remind you of the new strategies you aim to adopt, by taking it out and reading it carefully when you have a quiet moment in the day, and before you enter situations you know are likely to be problematic for you. At the same time, it would still be worth regularly going back to your detailed summary to remind you of the whole picture.

CHANGING THE RULES: MY SUMMARY

---

1. My old Rule is:

2. This Rule has had the following impact on my life:

3. I know that the Rule is in operation because:

---

4. It is understandable that I have this Rule, because:

5. However, the Rule is unreasonable, because:

6. The advantages of obeying the Rule are:

7. But the disadvantages are:

8. A more realistic and helpful Rule would be:

9. In order to test-drive the new Rule, I need to:

Dealing with the old Rule

Even when you have a well-formulated alternative and you are beginning to act on it, your old Rule may still rear its ugly head in the usual situations for a while. After all, it has been around for a long time and may not just slink quietly away as soon as you expose it to the light of day. If you are prepared for this, you will be able to tackle the old Rule calmly when you see it in operation, realising that this is a chance to deepen your new learning. This is where the work you did in Part Two, on anxious predictions and self-critical thoughts, will pay off. Remember that these are signs that your old Rule is in danger of being broken or has been broken. Keep using the core skills you learned in order to question your thoughts, find alternatives to them, and experiment with acting in different ways. Over time, you will find that you have less and less need to do so.

Experimenting with putting your new Rule into practice

As well as dealing with the old Rule when it turns up, it is important to develop a clear plan of action to help you experiment with acting in accordance with the new Rule and observing the outcome. Do the 'If . . . ' or 'Unless . . . ' and see if the 'then . . . ' follows. If you look back over Part Two, you may well find that in fact you have already been doing this when you checked out anxious thoughts, combated self-criticism by being kinder and fairer towards yourself, focused on your good points, gave yourself credit for your achievements, and treated yourself with care and respect. So, examine what you have already done and identify times when in fact you were putting your new Rule into practice even before you began to work on it in its own right.

In addition, ask yourself what else you need to do so as to ensure that your new Rule is indeed a useful policy and explore its impact on your everyday life. This means expanding your boundaries, discovering that it is still possible to feel good about yourself even if you are less than perfect, even if some people dislike and disapprove of you, even if you sometimes put yourself first, or even if you are sometimes gloriously out of control.

Make sure that you include specific changes in how you go about things, not just general strategies. Not just 'be more assertive', for example, but 'ask for help when I need it', 'say no when I disagree with someone', 'refuse requests when to carry them out would be very costly for me', 'be open about my thoughts and feelings with people I know well'. Then consider how to deliberately include these changes in your life. You could, for instance, use your **Daily Activity Diary** (see Part Two) to plan experiments at specific times, with specific people, in specific situations. Or you could use the **Experimenting with New Rules Worksheet** on pp. 311–17. There is another copy at the back of the book, which you can photocopy if you wish, and you will find it also at www.overcoming.co.uk.

Experimenting with New Rules Worksheet

Date/time	The situation	What I did	The outcome (what I noticed, felt, thought, learned)

Experimenting with New Rules Worksheet

Date/time	The situation	What I did	The outcome (what I noticed, felt, thought, learned)

Experimenting with New Rules Worksheet

Date/time	The situation	What I did	The outcome (what I noticed, felt, thought, learned)

Experimenting with New Rules Worksheet

Date/time	The situation	What I did	The outcome (what I noticed, felt, thought, learned)

Experimenting with New Rules Worksheet

Date/time	The situation	What I did	The outcome (what I noticed, felt, thought, learned)

Experimenting with New Rules Worksheet

Date/time	The situation	What I did	The outcome (what I noticed, felt, thought, learned)

Experimenting with New Rules Worksheet

Date/time	The situation	What I did	The outcome (what I noticed, felt, thought, learned)

Make sure you assess the results of your experiments, just as you did when you were checking out anxious predictions. Be specific – the clearer and more detailed the information you gather, the better. After each experiment, ask yourself:

- What are the signs that your new Rule is working?
- What are the signs that your new Rule is *not* working?
- What have you observed in yourself (e.g. your thoughts and feelings, your body state, changes in your behaviour) that tells you the new Rule is working (or not)?
- What have you seen in other people's reactions to you when you are following the new Rule?

Don't be surprised if acting in accordance with your new Rule feels uncomfortable at first. You may well feel quite apprehensive before you carry out experiments. If so, work out what you are predicting and use your experiment to check it out. (Remember to drop unnecessary precautions, otherwise you will not get the information you need.) Equally, you may find you feel guilty or worried after you have carried out an experiment, even if it has gone well. This happens, for example, with people who are experimenting with being less self-sacrificing or with dropping their standards from '110 per cent' to 'good enough'. Or again, you may get angry with yourself and become self-critical if you plan to carry out an experiment and then chicken out. If you experience uncomfortable feelings like these, look for the thoughts behind them and answer them, using the core skills you have already practised.

Be prepared

It could take as much as six to eight months for your new Rule to take over completely, so that you automatically operate from it without even needing to think about it. As long as it is useful to you and you can see it taking you in useful and interesting directions, don't give up. You may find it helpful to review your progress regularly and to set yourself targets. Ask yourself, for example:

- What have I achieved in the last week?
- What have I achieved in the last month?
- What do I want to aim for in the next week?
- What do I want to aim for in the next month?

Keeping written records of your experiments and their outcomes (whether on paper or electronically), and of unhelpful thoughts that you have tackled along the way, will help you to see how things are progressing. You can also look back over what you have done and use it as a source of encouragement, for example when things seem to be progressing slowly or your confidence has taken a knock.

Changing the Rules:
Written Summary – Rajiv

- *My old Rule is:*

  Unless I get it right, I will never get anywhere in life.

- *This Rule has had the following impact on my life:*

  I have always felt inadequate, not good enough. This has made me work tremendously hard, to the extent that I have been constantly under pressure, tense and stressed. This has affected my relationships. I have not had enough time for people, and I have lost out because of it. At times, it has made me quite ill.

  And I have sometimes run away from opportunities because I didn't think I would measure up.

- *I know the Rule is in operation because:*

  I get anxious about failing and put myself under more and more pressure. I go over the top in how I go about things – try to dot every 'i' and cross every 't'. I feel sick with anxiety. And if I think I've broken the Rule, I become very self-critical, get depressed, and give up altogether.

- *It is understandable that I have this Rule because:*

  When I was young, my father's disappointment with how his life has turned out made him very keen that we should all make the most of ourselves. Instead of encouraging and praising us, he gave us all the message that we were not up to it if we did not perform the way he wanted us to. That message sank in, and I have tried to compensate by being a perfectionist.

- *However, the Rule is unreasonable because:*

  It simply is not humanly possible to get it right all the time. Making mistakes and getting things wrong are all part of learning and growth.

- *The payoffs of obeying the Rule are:*

  Sometimes I do really good work, and get praise for it. This is partly why I have done so well in my career. People respect me. When I do get it right, I feel great.

- *But the disadvantages are:*

  I am constantly tense. Sometimes my work is not as good as it could be, because I get in such a state about it. I can't learn from my mistakes, because they upset me so much, nor can I learn from constructive criticism.

When things do not work out, I feel dreadful and it takes me ages to get over it. I avoid anything that I might not be able to get right, and miss all kinds of opportunities because of that. People may respect me, but it keeps them at a distance. They see me as a bit inhuman, unapproachable – even arrogant. The pressure I place on myself is bad for my health. Plus all my time and attention goes on my work – I don't allow myself to relax or do things I enjoy. In short, the Rule leads to stress, misery and fear on all fronts.

- *A more realistic and helpful new Rule would be:*

Good enough is good enough – I don't have to be great, to be great. I enjoy doing well – there's nothing wrong with that. But I'm only human and I will get it wrong sometimes. Getting it wrong is the route to growth.

- *In order to test-drive the new Rule, I need to:*
  - Keep reading this summary
  - Put my new Rule on a flashcard and on my mobile phone and read it several times a day
  - Cut my working hours and plan pleasures and social contact
  - Take time for myself
  - Revise my standards and give myself credit for less-than-perfect performance
  - Experiment with getting it wrong and observe the outcome. For example, practise sometimes saying 'I don't know' when people ask me questions
  - Plan my day in advance, and always plan less than I think I can do

- Focus on what I achieve, not on what I failed to do. Tomorrow is another day
- Remember: criticism can be useful – it doesn't mean I am a complete failure
- Watch out for signs of stress – they mean I am going back to my old ways
- Deal with the old pattern, when it comes up, using what I have learned to tackle anxious predictions and self-criticism

---

SUMMARY

1. When you have low self-esteem, unhelpful Rules for Living prevent you from getting what you want out of life and accepting yourself as you are.
2. Rules are learned through experience and observation. They are part of the culture we grow up in, and they are usually passed on to us by our families.
3. Many rules are helpful. But the unhelpful Rules for Living linked to low self-esteem are rigid, demanding and extreme, they restrict freedom of movement, and make change and growth difficult or impossible.
4. Rules are a way of coping with the apparent truth of your Bottom Line, but they do nothing to change it. In fact, they help to keep it in place.
5. Using the core skills you have already learned, you can learn to identify and change your unhelpful Rules, to question and re-think them, to create new Rules that are more realistic and give you more freedom to be yourself, and to experiment with testing them out in everyday life, until acting in accordance with them becomes second nature.

SECTION 2:

Creating a New Bottom Line

You have now laid the foundations for tackling your Bottom Line (the negative beliefs about yourself that underpin low self-esteem). Here is your chance to capitalise on all you have learned and to go to the heart of the matter. It could be that, after the work that you have done on your anxious and self-critical thoughts, on self-acceptance and on formulating new Rules for Living, your ideas about yourself have already changed – your Old Bottom Line may already look less convincing than it did. In this section, you will learn how to undermine your Old Bottom Line and how to create a new, more accepting and kinder alternative, once again using the core skills you have already practised (awareness, re-thinking and experiments).

You have, perhaps for many years, assumed that your Bottom Line reflects the real truth about you. Time now to take a fresh look. This section will help you to understand:

- how to identify your Old Bottom Line (Awareness)
- how to create a fairer, kinder and more compassionate New Bottom Line
- how to re-think the 'evidence' that appears to support your Old Bottom Line
- how to search for evidence that supports your New Bottom Line
- how to act on your New Bottom Line and carefully observe the outcome, to use experiments and observation to consolidate and strengthen it (Experiments)

How to identify your old Bottom Line (Awareness)

Having made your way through Parts One and Two, you may have already gained a pretty good idea of what your Bottom Line may be. Here are some possible sources of information that will help you to identify it more clearly:

1. Your knowledge of your own history
2. The fears expressed in your anxious predictions
3. Your self-critical thoughts
4. Thoughts that make it hard for you to focus on your good points, treat yourself kindly and enjoy life to the full
5. The imagined consequences of breaking your old Rules
6. The Downward Arrow (similar to what you used when identifying your Rule for Living in the last section, see p. 277)

Even if you are already pretty sure what your Bottom Line is, reviewing each source of information in turn will enable you to confirm your hunches, fine-tune the wording and perhaps discover other negative beliefs about yourself that you were less aware of. It is quite possible that you have more than one Bottom Line. If so, choose the Bottom Line that seems most important, and work on that. You can then use what you have learned to change other negative beliefs if you wish. Write down whatever hunches about your Bottom Line come to mind as you consider each potential source of information, even if you are not entirely sure of it.

1 Your knowledge of your own history

This draws on the work you did when you were puzzling out how your low self-esteem developed. When you read the people's stories in Part One, did any of them echo experiences you had when you were growing up? Even if they didn't, did you find yourself thinking back to when you were young and remembering things that happened to you and their effect on how you felt about yourself?

You can use these memories to clarify your Bottom Line. In particular, consider:

- What early experiences encouraged you to think badly of yourself? What events in your childhood and adolescence – or perhaps even later – led you to conclude that you were somehow lacking as a person?

_____

_____

_____

_____

_____

_____

- When did you first have this feeling about yourself? What images and memories come to mind when you are feeling anxious, or low, or bad about yourself? Do you remember specific events or incidents? Or was there a general atmosphere of unkindness, disapproval and criticism, or lack of affection?

_____

_____

_____

_____

_____

_____

- Whose voice do you hear when you are being hard on yourself? Whose face comes to mind? What messages did this person (or these people) give you about the kind of person you are?

_____

_____

_____

_____

_____

- What words were used to describe you when you failed to please or attracted criticism? (The words used by others may have become your own words for yourself.)

_____

_____

_____

_____

_____

2 The fears expressed in your anxious predictions

Think back to the work you did on your anxious predictions. Your fears, and the unnecessary precautions you took to keep yourself safe, may give you clues about your Bottom Line.

- Supposing what you most feared had come true. What would that have said about you as a person?

_____

_____

_____

_____

_____

- And what about your unnecessary precautions? What sort of person did you fear might be revealed if you did not take steps to conceal yourself?

_____

_____

_____

_____

_____

3 Your self-critical thoughts

Look back over the work you did on questioning your self-critical thoughts. These thoughts may be a direct reflection of your Bottom Line.

- What words did you use to describe yourself when you were being self-critical? What names did you call yourself? Look for repeating patterns. What negative beliefs about yourself might your self-critical thoughts reflect?

_____

_____

_____

_____

_____

- How similar are these words to words that were used about you by other people when you were small or when you were growing up?

_____

_____

_____

_____

_____

- When you do things that trigger self-criticism, what do those things suggest about you as a person? What sort of person would do things like that?

_____

_____

_____

_____

4 Thoughts that make it hard for you to accept your good points and positive qualities, treat yourself kindly and enjoy life to the full

Examine the doubts and reservations that came to mind when you were trying to list your good points and observe them in action in Part Two, Section 3.

- What thoughts made you reluctant to accept your good points and positive qualities as a true reflection of who you are?

_____

_____

_____

_____

_____

_____

- How did you disqualify or discount them?

_____

_____

_____

_____

_____

- What objections did you raise to giving yourself credit for your achievements, and treating yourself to relaxation and pleasure?

_____

_____

_____

_____

_____

- What beliefs about yourself might these doubts, reservations and disclaimers reflect?

_____

_____

---

5 The imagined consequences of breaking your old Rules

Go back to the Rules for Living that you identified in Section 1 of this Part (pp. 276–283) and look at what you imagined would happen if you broke them. Sometimes the imagined consequence is a more or less direct reflection of your Bottom Line (e.g. 'If I make a mistake, then *I am a failure*').

- If you break your Rules for Living, what does that say about you as a person?

- What kind of person makes mistakes, fails to win everyone's approval, loses their grip on their emotions, or whatever your Rules demand of you?

_____

_____

_____

- If your Rule takes the form of a 'should', would the 'or else' be a reflection of you as a person (e.g. 'I should always be constructively occupied [or else I am lazy]')?

_____

_____

_____

_____

_____

_____

6 The Downward Arrow

In Section 1, the Downward Arrow technique was explained as a way of identifying Rules for Living. It can also be used to identify your Bottom Line. The process is much the same as with Rules for Living, but the sequence of possible questions has a different emphasis and is designed to focus your attention on your negative beliefs about yourself, rather than your standards and expectations. You will see that the main change is to ask what each level of questioning _says about you_, rather than what it _means to you_ in terms of how you should behave and the sort of person you should be.

As before, the starting point is a vividly recalled specific incident where you felt bad about yourself. Rather than questioning particular thoughts, you then follow through a sequence of questions to help you identify what that situation says about you. You are looking here not for a particular self-critical thought occurring at a particular moment, but rather for something that is part of a pattern, something which pops into your mind over and over again, in many different situations, and has perhaps done so for many years. Let's take Briony, who we met in Part One, as an example. Here is a reminder of her story:

BRIONY'S STORY

Briony was adopted by her father's brother and his wife after her parents were killed in a car crash when she was seven. They already had two older daughters. Briony became the family scapegoat. Everything that went wrong was blamed on her. Briony was loving and liked to please people, but she faced new punishments every day no matter how hard she tried. She couldn't see friends, was made to give up music and was forced to do more than her fair share of work around the house.

One night, when she was eleven, Briony's stepfather came into her bedroom and raped her. He told her that she had asked for it, and that if she told anyone what had happened, no one would believe her. Afterwards, she crept around the house in terror. No one seemed to notice or care. Briony's doubts about herself crystallised into a firm belief at that point. She was bad. Other people could see it and would treat her accordingly.

And here is Briony's Downward Arrow, leading to her Bottom Line:

Situation:
New friend promised to phone and did not do so

Emotions:
Rejected, despairing

Body Sensations:
Sick to my stomach

Thought:
'He's forgotten'

If that was true, what would it mean about you?

'That I'm not worth remembering'

And what would that tell you about yourself?

'That he's backed off because he's seen the real me'

If he had, what would he have seen?

'Something he didn't like'

What would that be? What would he not like?

'The real me, that doesn't deserve to be liked or loved by anybody'

If that was true, what would it say about you as a person?

'I'm bad'

You can now use the 'Downward Arrow' technique to identify your own Bottom Line, using the worksheet on p. 334.

BOTTOM LINE DOWNWARD ARROW CHART

Situation:_____

Emotions: _____

Key thought:_____

What does that mean about me?

↓

_____

_____

↓

What does that mean about me?

↓

_____

_____

↓

What does that mean about me?

↓

_____

_____

↓

What does that mean about me?

↓

_____

_____

↓

So I am:

↓

_____

_____

As with Rules for Living, it may be helpful to use a range of different questions to find your Old Bottom Line, for example:

- Supposing that was true, what would it mean about me?
- Supposing that was true, what would it tell me about myself?
- What does that say about me as a person?
- What kind of person does that make me?
- What beliefs about myself does that reflect?
- What are the implications of that for how I see myself?

Remember that you are looking for an opinion about yourself that you have held over time and in many different situations. You may wish to confirm your findings (or have another go, if you are having trouble finding your Bottom Line, or putting it into words) by using a number of different situations in which you usually feel bad about yourself as your starting point.

Summarising your Old Bottom Line

Once you have a clear sense of what your Old Bottom Line is, write it down in your own words on the Bottom Line Worksheet on pp. 376–77. Then rate how far you believe it, from 0 to 100 per cent (100 per cent would mean that you still find it fully convincing; 50 per cent that you are in two minds; 5 per cent that you now hardly believe it at all, and so on).

If your self-esteem is relatively strong, your Bottom Line may only become convincing in particularly challenging situations. If so, make two ratings: first, how far you believe it when it is at its strongest, and second, how far you believe it when it is least convincing. Alternatively, you may find that your Bottom Line is more or less consistently present and convincing. In this case, you may need only one rating.

You may also find that your degree of belief has changed since you began to work on overcoming low self-esteem. If this is the case for you, record how far you believed your Bottom Line before you started the handbook, and how far you believe it now. Consider too what accounts for any changes you observe. Was it learning to face things that frightened you and discovering that the worst did not happen? Was it learning to escape the trap of self-critical thinking? Was it making the effort to focus on what is strong and good in yourself, and beginning to see yourself as someone who is worthy of kindness and compassion and deserves to enjoy life? Was it finding more flexible Rules for Living? Or perhaps some combination of these? If you can spot what helped, this will tell you what you need to continue doing for yourself.

How to create a new Bottom Line (Re-thinking)

Over time, you have probably accumulated a sizeable 'bank account' of negatively biased thoughts and memories that seem to support your Old Bottom Line. You can call on your 'Old Bottom Line Account' any time you want to, add new deposits, withdraw items and dwell on them like a miser counting and recounting money.

In contrast, creating a New Bottom Line opens an account in favour of yourself. It gives you a new place to store experiences that contradict your Old Bottom Line and support a fresh, kinder and more accepting perspective. You have somewhere you can deposit new ideas and experiences and keep them safe, knowing that they will be there for you when you need them.

The work you did in earlier parts may have given you some idea of what your New Bottom Line might be. As you checked out anxious predictions, questioned self-critical thoughts, focused on your good points, learned to be fair to yourself and to allow yourself to enjoy your life, as you changed your personal Rules, what new ideas about yourself came to mind?

- When you look back over all you have done in each of these areas, what do the changes you have made tell you about yourself? Are they entirely consistent with your old negative view?

_____

_____

_____

_____

_____

_____

- Do the qualities, strengths, assets and skills you have observed fit with your Old Bottom Line?

_____

_____

_____

_____

- Or do they suggest that it is a biased, unfair point of view that fails to take account of what is good and strong and worthy in you?

_____

_____

_____

_____

- What perspective on yourself would better account for *everything* you have observed?

_____

_____

_____

_____

_____

- What New Bottom Line would acknowledge that, like the rest of the human race, you are short of perfect, but that – along with your weaknesses and flaws – you have strengths and qualities, that it is fundamentally OK to be you?

_____

_____

_____

_____

_____

Your New Bottom Line may be the opposite of your Old Bottom Line (e.g. 'I am bad' ➤ 'I am good', or 'I am unworthy' ➤ 'I am worthy'). Or it may, so to speak, 'jump the tracks' and go off in a new direction which pretty much makes the Old Bottom Line irrelevant (e.g. 'I am worthless' ➤ 'I belong', or 'I am rubbish' ➤ 'I am a human being'). The key thing is to find a New Bottom Line that makes sense to you personally and holds the promise of changing how you feel about yourself.

IT'S WORTH REMEMBERING . . .

You are the judge and jury, not the counsel for the prosecution.

Your job is to take all the evidence into account, not just the evidence in favour of condemning the prisoner.

You may find that a New Bottom Line immediately springs to mind when you think back over everything you have done. Or your mind may be pretty much a blank, especially if your low self-esteem has been in place for a long time and you have a strong taboo on thinking well of yourself which still needs to be addressed.

Do not worry if this is the case. Your ideas will probably become clearer as you continue through the handbook. For the moment, it may be helpful to ask yourself: 'If I were not [your Old Bottom Line], what would I *really* like to be?' For example, 'If I were not incompetent, I would *really* like to be competent.'

Try this for yourself:

'If I were not _____

I would *really* like to be _____ '

If you can come up with an answer to the question, even if it seems pretty tentative and theoretical to you at the moment, record it. It will give you a good starting point for collecting evidence in favour of a new perspective. Conviction may come as you work through the chapter.

And bear in mind that, at this point, old ideas that it is wrong and big-headed to think well of yourself may surface – once again, 'yes, buts' may pop up. Remember that these are just old habits of thought, nothing more. You no longer have to listen to them, believe them, or do what they say.

Countering all-or-nothing thinking

As you know, this handbook is not about the power of positive thinking, or about encouraging you to become as unrealistically positive about yourself as you were unrealistically negative. It is about achieving a balanced, unbiased view of yourself, which puts your weaknesses and flaws in the context of a broadly favourable perspective and aims for 'good enough' rather than 'perfect', for the sense that it is OK to be you, just as you are.

Let us consider this in relation to the New Bottom Line 'I am likeable':

1. Imagine a line representing likeability:

0%   100%

Someone at the extreme right-hand end of the line would be 100 per cent likeable, while someone at the extreme left-hand end would be 0 per cent likeable.

2. Right now, put a cross on the line where you think you fall. If you have doubts about how likeable you are, you probably fall towards the left-hand end of the line.

Now consider what '0 per cent likeable' and '100 per cent likeable' actually mean.

In order to be '0 per cent likeable', you would have to be:	In order to be '100 per cent likeable', you would have to be:
• *Never* likeable, ever • *Completely* unlikeable (nothing about you could be at all likeable) • Not likeable to *anyone*	• Likeable *all the time* • *Completely* likeable (nothing about you could be at all unlikeable) • Likeable to *everyone*

Looking at it this way, you can probably see that to be 0 per cent or 100 per cent likeable is pretty much impossible. Nobody could be that dreadful – or that perfect.

3. Think now about someone you know. With the extremes (0 and 100 per cent) clearly in mind, where would you put him or her on the line?

_____

0%   100%

4. And, once again, keeping the extremes in mind, where would you now put yourself?

_____

0%   100%

When you decide on your New Bottom Line, keep this point in mind. You are not looking for the unattainable 100 per cent, you are looking for 'good enough'.

To check you are on the right track, it may be helpful at this point to return to the specific problem situation that was your starting point when you did the Downward Arrow to identify your existing Bottom Line. Once again, bring the situation vividly to mind, in high-definition detail. Then ask yourself: How would this situation have played out if the New Bottom Line I've come up with had been in place? Would things have been different in the way I would wish them to be? If the answer is yes, then continue to work with your first draft. If the answer is no, you may need to think again.

Summarising your New Bottom Line

When you have a sense of what it is, record your New Bottom Line on the Worksheet on pp. 376–7. Rate how far you believe it,

341

just as you rated your belief in your Old Bottom Line, including variations in how convincing it seems to you and how your belief has changed since you began to work on overcoming your low self-esteem. Then take a moment to focus your attention on it and note what emotions and body sensations come up and how strong they are. As you continue through the handbook, come back to this summary from time to time, and observe how your belief in your New Bottom Line changes as you focus on evidence that supports and strengthens it.

Don't worry if, for the moment, your belief in your New Bottom Line is low. If your Old Bottom Line has been in place for a long time, it will take patience, persistence and practice to make the new one powerfully convincing. Let us now move on to consider how to undermine your Old Bottom Line further, and how to strengthen the New Bottom Line you have tentatively identified.

What evidence appears to support your Old Bottom Line?

Your negative beliefs about yourself are based on experience – an attempt to make sense of what has happened to you. This means that, as you look back over your life, you are likely to see lots of 'evidence' that seems to support them. Remember that, thanks to biased thinking, you are likely to have noticed and remembered what seemed to support your negative beliefs, and to have screened out or discounted what did not. Examining this so-called 'evidence' – and searching for other ways to explain it – is the next step towards overcoming low self-esteem.

What sources of 'evidence' might seem to support your Old Bottom Line?

Reflect for a moment on your Old Bottom Line and ask yourself:

- What experiences, past and present, come to mind?
- What events appear to support it?
- What makes you say that you are inadequate, unlovable, incompetent, or whatever your Bottom Line may be?
- What leads you to reach such negative conclusions about yourself?

Supporting 'evidence' varies from person to person. Sometimes most of it is found in the past, in relationships or experiences. However, more recent events can also be used as sources of evidence. Some common sources are listed, with examples, below. Which of these ring bells for you?

COMMON SOURCES OF 'EVIDENCE'

1. Current difficulties and symptoms of distress
2. Failure to overcome current difficulties without help
3. Past errors and failures
4. Specific shortcomings
5. Physical characteristics
6. Psychological characteristics
7. Differences between yourself and other people
8. Other people's behaviour towards you, past or present
9. The behaviour of others for whom you feel responsible
10. Loss of something that was a part of your identity

Use this section as an opportunity to reflect on the sources of 'evidence' you are using to support your Old Bottom Line. Tick the ones you recognise.

1 Current difficulties and symptoms of distress

People with low self-esteem may have a range of difficulties and symptoms. For example, low self-esteem might sometimes make you feel quite depressed. You may then find it hard to gear yourself up to do anything. This could make you see yourself as lazy. In other words, you might see your depression as yet another sign of what a bad person you are, rather than a temporary symptom of an understandable state, which will disappear once your mood lifts.

Does this sound familiar? ☐

2 Failure to overcome current difficulties without help

You might see being unable to manage independently as a sign of weakness or failure. This could have prevented you from asking for the support you needed from partners, relatives or friends. Yet two heads are sometimes better than one. Talking things through with someone who knows us well can help to free up our own thinking, and the fact is that everybody needs help and support in life, especially when times are tough.

Does this sound familiar? ☐

3 Past errors and failures

From time to time, we all do things we regret. We can all be selfish, thoughtless, irritable, or less than fully honest. We all take short cuts, make mistakes, avoid challenges and fail to achieve objectives. Perhaps you would see such actions as evidence of basic inadequacy rather than normal human weakness?

Does this sound familiar? ☐

4 Specific shortcomings

No one is perfect. We all have aspects of ourselves that we would like to change or improve. Perhaps you see these shortcomings as further proof that there is something fundamentally wrong with

344

you, rather than as specific problems which have developed for a reason, and which it might in fact be possible to resolve?

Does this sound familiar? ☐

5 Physical characteristics

You may feel that you are too tall, too short, too fat, too thin, the wrong skin colour, the wrong shape or the wrong build. And you might use these observations to undermine your sense of self-esteem. For instance, someone who sees themselves as overweight might feel completely fat, ugly and unattractive. They would probably ignore all the other things that made them attractive, such as their sense of style, their ability to enjoy life and their intelligence.

Does this sound familiar? ☐

6 Psychological characteristics

Psychological characteristics – especially those that have attracted criticism in childhood (such as having a high energy level or being strong-willed) – might lead you to feel bad about yourself. Instead of seeing your qualities as gifts, you might see them as further evidence that you are unacceptable to others. Similarly, people who do not conform to cultural or family stereotypes (such as gender stereotypes) may feel this means there is something wrong with them, rather than with the over-rigid expectations of others.

Does this sound familiar? ☐

7 Differences between yourself and other people

However talented you are, there are probably other people who are more talented. However much you have, there are probably others who have more. People with low self-esteem sometimes compare themselves unfavourably with other people they know, or with images from the popular press or social media. Perhaps you use comparisons with other people as a source of evidence to support your poor opinion of yourself?

Does this sound familiar? ☐

8 Other people's behaviour towards you, past or present

People who were treated badly as children may see this treatment as evidence of their own lack of worth, whether the treatment came from family, schoolmates or the society in which they lived. Equally, dislike, rejection, disapproval or abuse in the present can help to create or reinforce low self-esteem.

Does this sound familiar? ☐

9 The behaviour of others for whom you feel responsible

This is a particular trap for people with low self-esteem who become parents. They may blame themselves for anything that goes wrong in their children's lives, even long after the children have grown up and left home.

Does this sound familiar? ☐

10 Loss of something that was a part of your identity

As we said in Section 1 of this part of the handbook (p. 268), people hang their self-esteem on a range of different pegs, such as wealth, career or relationships. If the peg on which you have hung your sense of worth is taken away (for instance, if you lose your job), this may expose you to the full force of negative beliefs about yourself. It may be taken as another sign that you are not good enough, even if there are several other convincing reasons for it (e.g. the company was doing badly and had to make some cutbacks).

Does this sound familiar? ☐

How else can the 'evidence' be understood?

Each source of 'evidence' that you used to support your Old Bottom Line is open to different interpretations. Once you have identified the evidence that you feel backs up your Old Bottom Line, your next task is to examine it carefully and assess how far it truly supports what you have been in the habit of believing about yourself (re-thinking). Make a note of your conclusions on the Bottom Line Worksheet at the end of this section if you wish.

You may find the following questions useful. You will see that they relate directly to the various sources of evidence outlined above. It may also be worth bearing in mind the questions you used to tackle self-critical thoughts in Part Two.

KEY QUESTIONS

When Reviewing the 'Evidence' for Your Old Bottom Line

1. Aside from personal inadequacy, what other explanations could there be for current difficulties or signs of distress?
2. Although it is useful to be able to manage independently, what might be the advantages of being able to ask for help and support?
3. How fair is it to judge yourself on the basis of past errors and failures?
4. How fair is it to judge yourself on the basis of specific shortcomings?
5. How helpful is it to let your self-esteem depend on rigid ideas about what you should do or be?
6. Just because someone is better at something than you, or has more than you do, does that make them better as a person?

---

7. What reasons, besides the kind of person you are, might there be for others' behaviour towards you?
8. How much power do you actually have over the behaviour of people you feel responsible for?
9. What aspects of yourself could you value and appreciate, aside from what you have lost?

1 Aside from personal inadequacy, what other explanations could there be for current difficulties or signs of distress?

If this is a time when you are having difficulties or experiencing distress, rather than taking this as a sign that there is something fundamentally wrong with you, look at what is going on in your life at the moment.

• Is anything happening that might make sense of how you are feeling?

_____

_____

_____

• If someone you cared about was going through what you are going through right now, might they feel similar?

_____

_____

_____

_____

- How would you react to them? Would you assume that they, too, must be inadequate, bad or whatever?

_____

_____

_____

_____

- Or would you consider their reactions to be understandable, given what was going on, and respond to them with compassion?

_____

_____

_____

_____

- Even if nothing very obvious is happening in your life right now to explain how you feel, how far could it be understood in terms of old habits of thinking which are a result of your past experiences? If so, what if you were able to be kind to yourself, to be more encouraging and supportive?

_____

_____

_____

_____

2 Although it is useful to be able to manage independently, what might be the advantages of being able to ask for help and support?

You may feel that asking for help is a sign of weakness, and that you should be able to stand on your own two feet. But perhaps being able to ask for help when you genuinely need it actually puts you in a stronger position, not a weaker one, because it may give you a chance to deal successfully with a wider range of situations than you could manage on your own.

- How do you feel when other people who are in difficulties come to you for help or support?

_____

_____

_____

_____

_____

- Do you automatically conclude that they must be feeble or pathetic? If not, how do you react?

_____

_____

_____

_____

- Have you ever felt useful, wanted and warm towards another person because you were able to offer them help? Maybe this is how other people who care about you would feel about you, if you gave them half a chance?

_____

_____

_____

_____

Alternatively, you may fear that if you ask for help, you will be disappointed. Other people may refuse, or be scornful, or not be able to give you what you need. It makes sense to select people who you have no strong evidence to suppose will react in this way. That aside, the best way to test out how others will react is to try it – to experiment. Work out your predictions in advance and check them out, just as you learned to do in Part Two.

3 How fair is it to judge yourself on the basis of past errors and failures?

People with low self-esteem sometimes confuse what they _do_ with what they _are_. They assume that a bad action is a sign of a bad person, or that failing at something means being a failure through and through. If this were true, no one in the world could ever feel good about themselves. We may regret things we have done, but it is not helpful or accurate to move on from that to complete self-condemnation.

- Do you believe that you are thoroughly bad, worthless, inadequate or useless, because of something you did in the past?

_____

_____

_____

_____

- What if, instead, you could see your past failings in terms of natural human error, or a product of your experiences?

_____

_____

_____

This is not the same as letting yourself off the hook. It is a first step towards putting right whatever needs to be put right and thinking about how you might avoid making the same mistakes in future. What you did may have been the only thing you could have done, given your circumstances and your state of knowledge at the time. Now you can see things differently, so you can take advantage of your broader current perspective. And remember: you may have done a bad or stupid thing, but that does not make you a bad or stupid person.

4 How fair is it to judge yourself on the basis of specific shortcomings?

Having something about yourself that you would like to improve makes you part of the human race.

- Maybe you have difficulty asserting yourself, or being punctual, or organising your time, or talking to people without anxiety. How does it follow that there is something fundamentally wrong with you as a person?

_____

_____

_____

_____

- How would you judge another person with the same specific difficulty?

_____

_____

_____

- If your reaction to another person would be different, then what if you took a kinder and more accepting approach to yourself?

_____

_____

_____

Bear in mind that your shortcomings, whatever they are, are only one side of you (remember your list of positive qualities and good points). And after all, you are just another normal, fallible human being.

5 How helpful is it to let your self-esteem depend on rigid ideas about what you should do or be?

You may have always been aware that your self-esteem was based on a particular aspect of yourself (e.g. your ability to make people laugh, your physical strength, or your capacity to earn a high salary). Or you may have only recognised what you depended on after you had lost it (e.g. perhaps you are ageing, your physical beauty has faded, you have retired, or your family has left home).

- What does your worth depend on, _apart from_ the one thing you have decided is your be-all and end-all?

_____

_____

_____

_____

- How many of the qualities, strengths, skills and talents on your list of positive qualities depend on the peg you usually hang your self-esteem on?

_____

_____

_____

_____

- Think about people you know, like and respect. What attracts you to them? When you consider why you value each person, how important is the one thing your own self-esteem depends on?

_____

_____

_____

_____

_____

6 Just because someone is better at something than you, or has more than you do, does it make them better than you as a person?

The fact that some people are more beautiful, more competent, richer or more advanced in their careers does not make them any better than you as people.

- How possible is it for anyone to be best at everything?

_____

_____

_____

_____

- What might be the benefits of judging each person on their own merits?

_____

_____

_____

_____

- How would it be if you had a sense of your own worth, regardless of how you stand in relation to other people, or to the idealised images promoted by the popular press and social media?

_____

_____

_____

_____

_____

7 What reasons, besides the kind of person you are, might there be for others' behaviour towards you?

People with low self-esteem often assume that if others treat them badly or react to them negatively, this must in some way be deserved. This can make it difficult to set limits to what you will allow others to do to you, to feel entitled to others' time and attention, to assert your own needs, and to end relationships that damage you.

There are many possible reasons why people behave as they do. In the case of the particular person (or people) whose behaviour seems to you to back up your Old Bottom Line, ask yourself: what other reasons could there be for what they do?

- What, in their own early experiences, might have made it difficult for them to behave any differently (just as children who are abused or treated violently often become abusers or violent themselves)?

_____

_____

_____

- What might there be, in their current circumstances, that is prompting them to behave badly (e.g. stress, pressure, illness, fear)?

_____

_____

_____

- Is it possible that, without them necessarily being aware of it, you remind them of someone they do not get on with?

_____

_____

_____

- Is it possible that you are simply not their cup of tea?

_____

_____

_____

- How far do they behave in the same way with others? Perhaps there is nothing personal about the way they treat you – their manner is critical or sharp or dismissive with everyone, not just with you?

_____

_____

_____

If you find it difficult to detach yourself from your usual self-blaming perspective and to think of other reasons why people behave towards you as they do, consider how you explain bad behaviour or unkindness towards people other than yourself. For example:

- When a case of child abuse is reported in the newspapers, who do you immediately assume is to blame – the child? Or the adult abuser?

_____

_____

_____

- Similarly, if you read about intimidation, persecution, rape or assault, who do you hold responsible for that? Do you automatically conclude that the person on the receiving end must have deserved it? Or can you see that the perpetrator is responsible for what he or she did?

_____

_____

_____

- What about civilian victims of war? Do you consider that they are to blame for their fate? Or do you see them as innocent victims of violence carried out by others for their own reasons?

_____

_____

_____

In each of these cases, do you always assume that it must in some way be the fault of the person who is treated badly? Or do you explain what happened in some other way? If so, try applying similar more compassionate explanations to your own experiences.

8 How much power do you actually have over the behaviour of people you feel responsible for?

It's important to remember that we usually have very limited power over other people's behaviour.

- For instance, if you have a dinner party, you can provide good food and drink, and you can ask a mix of people who you think will get on with one another – but how far can you guarantee that everyone will enjoy themselves?

_____

_____

_____

_____

- Likewise, how far can you prevent a teenage child from going out with friends you think are a bad influence (without forbidding your son or daughter from leaving the house and completely removing the independence they need as a young adult)?

_____

_____

_____

Try to be clear about the limits of your responsibility towards other people. There are some things you can realistically do to influence them (such as talking to them in a calm, caring way). But there are other things (such as what they do when they are elsewhere) that are beyond your control. It is reasonable partly to base your good opinion of yourself on your willingness to meet your responsibilities. It is not reasonable to base your self-esteem on things over which you have no control.

9 What aspects of yourself could you value and appreciate, aside from what you have lost?

- Look back at the work you did on appreciating your strong points and qualities (Part Two, Section 3). What aspects of yourself could counterbalance your sense that the peg you have hung your self-esteem on is lost?

_____

_____

_____

_____

- Think about people you like, love and respect. What is it about them that you appreciate, apart from the one thing that you have based your own self-esteem on?

_____

_____

_____

_____

Summarising the evidence for your Old and New Bottom Lines

Here is how Briony summarised the experiences that seemed to support her Old Bottom Line ('I am bad'), and how she now understood them after carefully thinking things through and formulating a New Bottom Line ('I am worthy').

'EVIDENCE' FOR OLD BOTTOM LINE	NEW UNDERSTANDING
My parents died – blamed myself.	They loved me dearly and would never have left me if they could have helped it.
My step-parents' behaviour.	Not my fault – their behaviour was vicious and cruel, and there was no reason for it. No child deserves to be treated like that.

My stepfather's abuse.	It was a wicked thing to do. He knew it: that is why he concealed it. He was the adult; I was the child. He should never have abused my trust like that. It was sick.
My first marriage – husband ridiculed and criticised me, wore me down.	I now know he was like that in other relationships. Given what had already happened to me, I was in no position to fight back. My belief that I was bad made me think I deserved it.
People being irritable or unkind or putting me down.	Bound to happen sometimes – can't please everyone. Does not mean I am bad.

In the light of this new understanding, Briony now believed her Old Bottom Line: 30 per cent (as opposed to 100 per cent when she first started the handbook).

In the light of this new understanding, Briony now believed her New Bottom Line: 55 per cent (as opposed to 0 per cent).

Now (using the Bottom Line Worksheet at the end of the section if you wish) complete your own summary of the experiences that have seemed to support your Old Bottom Line, and of how you now understand them. Notice if there is any change in how far you believe your New and Old Bottom lines. If so, what made the difference? If not, it may be worth taking another look at your 'evidence' for the Old Bottom Line. But first of all, it's time to take a closer look at the New Bottom Line.

The other side of the story: What evidence supports your New Bottom Line?

There are two main ways of collecting new evidence that supports your New Bottom Line and contradicts the old one: observation and experiments. (If you have not yet defined a New Bottom Line you are comfortable with, stick with looking for evidence which is not consistent with your Old Bottom Line.)

Observation

Part One described how your Old Bottom Line is kept in place by negative biases in perception and interpretation. These make it easy for you to notice information that supports your Old Bottom Line, while encouraging you to screen out information that contradicts it. You worked on correcting this bias when you made your list of good points and positive qualities and set about recording examples of them in your behaviour. A good starting point now is to review your list and your records and highlight anything that contradicts your old, self-critical Bottom Line. Don't forget the fact that you are working your way through this handbook; it is a reflection of your courage, persistence and resourcefulness.

The next step is actively to seek out and record information which directly contradicts your old ideas about yourself and supports and strengthens a new, more generous perspective. The information (or evidence) you need to look for will depend on the exact nature of your Bottom Line. If, for example, your Old Bottom Line was 'I am unlikeable' and your New Bottom Line is 'I am likeable', then you will need to collect evidence that supports the idea that you are indeed likeable (for example, people smiling at you, people wanting to spend time with you, or people saying that they enjoy your company). If, on the other hand, your Old Bottom Line was 'I am incompetent' and your New Bottom Line is 'I am competent', then you will need to collect evidence that supports the idea that you are indeed competent (for example, meeting deadlines, responding sensibly to questions, or handling crises at work effectively).

In order to find out what information you personally need to look for, make a list of as many things as you can think of in answer to the following questions:

• What experiences (evidence) would you see as inconsistent with your Old Bottom Line?

_____

_____

_____

_____

• What information or experiences would suggest to you that your Old Bottom Line is inaccurate, unfair or invalid?

_____

_____

_____

_____

• Conversely, what evidence would you see as consistent with your New Bottom Line?

_____

_____

_____

_____

- What information or experiences would suggest to you that your New Bottom Line is accurate, fair and valid?

_____

_____

_____

_____

Make sure the items on your list are absolutely clear and specific. If they are vague and poorly defined, you will have trouble deciding whether you have observed them or not.

Again, let's take Briony's summary of evidence supporting her New Bottom Line as an example.

Evidence from Briony's past is:

- My parents loved me. I know that from my own memories and from photos and things I have.
- My grandmother loved me. She couldn't protect me, but she made me feel worthwhile and lovable.
- I made some friends at school, though I was too prickly and unhappy to have many (not my fault).
- Even when I was being abused in my first marriage, I managed to hold down a job, and then, after having the children, I protected them from their father. When he began to show signs of abusing them I got up the courage to leave, even though I never thought I would make it alone.
- I found a second husband who loves and supports me. He is a good man, and he chose me and stuck by me in spite of all my difficulties.
- I have struggled to overcome what happened to me and made a good fist of it.
- All the good points on my list.

Evidence from Briony's present life is:

- Things I do for other people.
- Things I contribute to society (e.g. my charity work and political activism).
- My good points, day to day (from list).
- My relationships – signs that people love me (e.g. phone calls, letters, invitations, people stopping to talk to me).

In the light of this evidence, Briony now believed her Old Bottom Line: 20 per cent

In the light of this evidence, Briony now believed her New Bottom Line: 85 per cent

Now use the Bottom Line Worksheet at the end of the section to complete your own summary of evidence from the past and from the present that supports your New Bottom Line, and rate how far you now believe both your Old and your New Bottom Lines.

Experiments

Now is the time to push back the walls of the prison that low self-esteem has built around you, by experimenting with acting as if your New Bottom Line was true, daring to break out and begin to move more freely and extend your range. If you wish, you could use the **Acting in Accordance with my New Bottom Line** worksheet (p. 373) to record what you do and the outcome of your experiments.

Despite the work you have already done on re-thinking your Old Bottom Line, you may still feel uncomfortable or even fearful of doing this. This is hardly surprising. If your Old Bottom Line was not well embedded and compelling, you would have escaped its clutches long ago. Notice what thoughts run through your mind when you consider entering new situations, and perhaps also when you have succeeded in being your new self and then afterwards begin to doubt how well it went. The chances are you will find anxious predictions and self-critical thoughts behind these feelings. If so, you know how to tackle them. Now fill in this section on the worksheet on pp. 376–7.

Once again, the experiments you need to carry out depend on the exact nature of your New Bottom Line. Ask yourself:

• What experiences would confirm and strengthen your new perspective on yourself?

_____

_____

_____

_____

• What do you need to do in order to discover whether this new perspective is useful and rings true?

_____

_____

_____

_____

• You experimented in Part Two with approaching what you usually avoided and dropping your unnecessary precautions – how does what you discovered fit here?

_____

_____

_____

_____

- What other experiments could you carry out on similar lines?

_____

_____

_____

_____

- Equally, consider the changes you made in Part Two, Section 3, when you were learning to treat yourself kindly and build rewards into your life. How do *those* fit with what you are doing now?

_____

_____

_____

_____

- Are there other similar things you could do now to strengthen your belief in your New Bottom Line?

_____

_____

_____

_____

- What would someone who believed your New Bottom Line do, on a day-to-day basis?

_____

_____

_____

_____

For example, to strengthen her 'I am worthy' Bottom Line, Briony decided to improve her social life by:

- Making the first approach to people she trusted, rather than waiting for them to contact her
- Gradually being more open about herself with people
- Planning treats and pleasures for herself

Make a list of as many experiments as you can think of in different areas of life, under the following headings:

Work
Leisure time

Close relationships

Social life

Looking after yourself

Here are some more examples, to give you some ideas:

If you are usually a perfectionist about your work, try . . .

- Dropping your standards and spending less time preparing reports and documents
- Going for 'good enough'

If you usually worry about your weight, try . . .

- Wearing brightly coloured, stylish clothes instead of trying to fade into the wallpaper
- Eating something you enjoy, with relish

If you usually rehearse everything before you say it, try . . .

- Saying the first thing that comes into your head
- Showing what you really feel about something

If you are usually apologetic about asking people for anything, try . . .

- Acting as if you were entitled to time and attention
- Asking for help even when you don't really need it

If you usually agree to do things for other people in order to get their approval, try . . .

- Saying 'no'
- Doing something just for yourself

If you usually avoid talking about your feelings, try . . .

- Asking a friend for help when something upsets you
- Showing someone how much you like them

When you have a list of specific experiments, covering all these aspects of your life, transfer them to the Worksheet on p. 376 which summarises your work on your Bottom Line. And then begin to put them into practice in your daily life.

Here is Briony's summary, as an example:

Observation: Information and experiences I need to be alert to, in order to gather more evidence to support my New Bottom Line

- Things I do for other people, especially all the time and care I put into the children. My love for them, and for my husband. The pleasure I take in them. My creativity and imagination in looking after them and helping them to develop into good people.
- Things I contribute to society (my charity work, my political activism).
- My good points as they show themselves day to day.
- My relationships – signs that people love me – phone calls, letters, invitations, people stopping to talk to me and wanting me to get involved in things.
- My intelligence – at last I am starting to think I am worth educating and am doing something about it.

Experiments: Specific things I need to do, in order to gather more evidence to support my New Bottom Line

- Begin making the first approach to people I trust, rather than leaving it up to them.
- Gradually be more open about myself with people and see if they really do back off.
- Plan treats and pleasures for myself – I deserve it.
- Make time to study. Start saving for a proper course.
- Give more responsibility to the others at home to keep the show on the road.
- Look for a better job, one that really uses what I have got to offer.

Assessing the outcome of your experiments

Make sure that you assess the outcome of your experiments carefully, just as you assessed the outcome of your experiments when you checked out your anxious predictions in Part Two. Keeping a careful record of your observations and your experiments, exactly what you did and how it turned out, will help you to collect and remember information to support your New Bottom Line. Experiment by experiment, keep asking yourself: How far do I now believe both my Old and my New Bottom Lines? The more you act on your new perspective the stronger it will become, especially if you stay open-minded and curious and willing to have a go and learn. Remember: direct experience is the best teacher.

You will find worksheets to help you do this on pp. 373–375. There is also a blank worksheet, which you can photocopy if you wish, on p. 450 or you can download the worksheet at www. overcoming.co.uk.

Acting in Accordance with my New Bottom Line

Date/Time	Experiment (what I did)	Results (what I noticed, my feelings, sensations and thoughts, others' reactions, what I learned)	My belief in my Old Bottom Line	My belief in my New Bottom Line

Acting in Accordance with my New Bottom Line

Date/Time	Experiment (what I did)	Results (what I noticed, my feelings, sensations and thoughts, others' reactions, what I learned)	My belief in my Old Bottom Line	My belief in my New Bottom Line

Acting in Accordance with my New Bottom Line

Date/Time	Experiment (what I did)	Results (what I noticed, my feelings, sensations and thoughts, others' reactions, what I learned)	My belief in my Old Bottom Line	My belief in my New Bottom Line

BOTTOM LINE WORKSHEET

When you have rated your degree of belief, take a moment to focus on your Bottom Line and notice what feelings emerge. Write down any emotions you experience (e.g. sadness, anger, guilt), and rate them according to how powerful they are (from 0 to 100). Again, you may notice that, although you can still call up your Bottom Line, your feelings when you focus on it are less intense.

My Old Bottom Line is: 'I am _____
_____ ,

	Belief	Emotions (0–100)
When the Old Bottom Line is most convincing:	_____	%
When it is least convincing:	_____	%
When I started the book:	_____	%

My New Bottom Line is: 'I am _____
_____ ,

	Belief	Emotions (0–100)
When the New Bottom Line is most convincing:	_____	%
When it is least convincing:	_____	%
When I started the book:	_____	%

'Evidence' supporting the Old Bottom Line and how I now understand it:

'Evidence'   **New Understanding**

In the light of my new understanding,
  I now believe my Old Bottom Line: _____ %
In the light of my new understanding,
  I now believe my New Bottom Line: _____ %

Evidence (past and present) which supports my New
Bottom Line:

_____

_____

_____

_____

_____

In the light of this evidence,
   I now believe my Old Bottom Line: _____ %
In the light of this evidence,
   I now believe my New Bottom Line: _____ %

Observation: Information and experiences I need to be
alert to, in order to gather more evidence to support my
New Bottom Line:

_____

_____

_____

_____

_____

_____

Experiments: Specific things I need to do, in order to
gather more evidence to support my New Bottom Line:

_____

_____

_____

_____

_____

Creating and strengthening a New Bottom Line does not happen overnight. It may take weeks (or even months) of observation and experimentation before you find your New Bottom Line fully convincing. You have accumulated a lifetime of 'evidence' that supports your Old Bottom Line, stored it and mulled it over. You will not need a similar lifetime of evidence in support of your New Bottom Line – that would be rather discouraging! But you should expect to make some investment in time and energy, some regular commitment to record-keeping and practice, in order to reach the point where thinking and acting in accordance with your New Bottom Line become second nature. When you reach this point, you have made the final step towards accepting and valuing yourself just as you are. The last section of the handbook will give you some ideas on how to reach this point.

SUMMARY

1. Your final step towards overcoming low self-esteem is to identify your old, negative Bottom Line in your own words. You can use a number of different sources of information to become aware of it and bring it into focus.

2. Then you are ready to formulate a kinder, fairer and more balanced alternative – a New Bottom Line. This sets the scene for you to begin noticing and recording information you have previously screened out, which contradicts your old beliefs about yourself.

3. The next step is to identify the 'evidence' you have used to support your Old Bottom Line, and to search for other ways of understanding it – rather than assuming that it must reflect the real truth about you (re-thinking).

4. Finally, time for experiments. Decide what experiences and information would support your New Bottom Line and begin to seek them out, both by observation and by acting as if your New Bottom Line was true and observing the results.

SECTION 3:

Planning for the Future

Introduction

In working through this handbook, you have tackled the various thinking habits that keep low self-esteem going. You have created new Rules for Living and a new Bottom Line and worked out how to put them into practice and act as if they were true on a day-to-day basis. In this section, the practical ideas for overcoming low self-esteem that you have been working with will be related back to the flowcharts introduced in Part One, which mapped out how low self-esteem develops and what keeps it going in the present day (pp. 23 and 54). That way, you will be able to see how what you have been doing fits with the understanding of low self-esteem that was your starting point. We shall then move on to consider ways of ensuring that the changes you have made are consolidated and carried forward, rather than left behind when you close the handbook.

Old habits die hard. Particularly at times when you are stressed, or when you are feeling low or unwell, your Old Bottom Line may surface again, and – along with it – your old habits of expecting the worst and criticising yourself may begin to re-establish themselves.

There is no need to worry about this. Long-established habits of thinking are probably never deleted from the brain's 'hard disk'. So given the right circumstances, they may well pop up again. But now things are different. You know what to do, how to break the vicious circle that keeps low self-esteem going, and you have established new

Rules for Living and a New Bottom Line and repeatedly put them into practice. So, you are no longer stuck with only one unkind and painful point of view – you have somewhere else to go. It is simply a question of going back to what you already know and practising it systematically until you have got yourself back on an even keel. If you have a healthy awareness that a setback could occur, you will be in a good position to spot early warning signs that your Old Bottom Line is resurfacing and to deal with it without delay. You may be able to put it back in its place almost immediately, or it may take you a little time.

Either way, even if unpleasant, this will be a valuable opportunity for learning, a chance to become more sensitive to early warning signals that all is not well, and to discover again that the new ideas and skills you have acquired can work for you. By planning ahead and considering how setbacks might come about, you will ensure that the changes you have made will last in the long term.

This section will help you to:

- update your understanding of your low self-esteem
- draft an Action Plan for the future, using Key Questions and SMART criteria
- fine-tune your Action Plan so that it has the best chance of being helpful to you

Updating your understanding of your low self-esteem

The flowcharts on pp. 385 and 387 explain the development and persistence of low self-esteem. You are already familiar with this, from Parts One and Two. You will see that here we have used the flowcharts to summarise the different methods you have learned to use as you have made your way through the handbook, to re-think unhelpful old thinking patterns, change your Rules, undermine your Old Bottom Line, and establish and strengthen your New

Bottom Line. This is so that you can see clearly how the changes you have made fit together in a coherent plan for overcoming low self-esteem.

Following the flowcharts on pp. 385 and 387, you will find blank versions with just the headings, and space left for you to write. These are also available at www.overcoming.co.uk. Here is your opportunity to review and update the work you did earlier (in Part One, Sections 2 and 3), when you charted a personal picture of the development and persistence of your low self-esteem. You may find that the picture now is much the same, or you may find that working on your anxious and self-critical thoughts, on enhancing self-acceptance, and on creating new Rules for Living and a New Bottom Line, has helped you to understand more fully the story of your low self-esteem. You can use the flowcharts to summarise your up-to-date understanding of how the problem came into being, and what kept it going.

Drafting an Action Plan

The point of an Action Plan is to have something which you can easily review and refer to when you need it, for example to check your progress or to remind you how to manage a setback. This means that:

- **It must be easy to find**, whether on paper or electronic. If you cannot find your Action Plan, you will not be able to make use of it. Leaving it lying around to get stained and dog-eared, or buried in some obscure part of your computer or phone is like sending a message to yourself that it doesn't really matter – *your future* doesn't really matter. So, make sure that you look after your Action Plan. You need to know where it is and be able to find it easily when you need it. Decide right now where you want to keep it. Put it somewhere special, if you can: somewhere that is yours and yours alone.

- **It must be short**. Your Action Plan will be most helpful to you if it is not too long. If there are points you want to go into in more detail, put them on separate sheets and staple them to the Action Plan worksheets in this handbook. And if there are particular parts of the handbook that you want to be able to come back to easily, get some coloured Post-It notes and stick them in the book so that these parts are easy to identify.

Your Action Plan – The first draft

In a form that makes it easy to edit, change and improve, write down your answers to the questions you will find on p. 393, using the worksheets on pp. 396–404. As you go along, make a note of any other helpful points that occur to you. This is the first draft of your Action Plan. Think of solidly grounded, healthy self-esteem as your marker on the horizon. Your learning summary and action plan are the kit you need in your backpack to support you on your continuing journey.

When you have completed your first draft, review it and see if you have left out anything important. To refresh your memory of everything you have done, go back through all three parts of the handbook, including what you have written on the charts and worksheets. When you are satisfied that you have the best possible version for the time being, put your Action Plan into practice for two or three weeks. Remind yourself regularly of what it says and keep it at the back of your mind, so that you can capitalise on any useful experiences that come up. You may find it helpful to give yourself some simple reminder cues – sticky coloured dots in places you can easily see them for instance, or reminders on your smartphone.

Your Action Plan – The second draft

After two or three weeks of putting your first draft into practice, you should have a good idea of how helpful your Action Plan is. Now is a good time to review it and refine it, if you wish. You may find that you have left out something vital, or that what seemed clear to you when you wrote it down seems less helpful when you try to apply it in real life.

Make whatever changes seem necessary, and then write out a revised version for a longer test-drive. Decide for yourself how long you will practise applying this version – perhaps three months? Or six months? This will give you an opportunity to find out how helpful the plan is in the longer term, how well established your New Bottom Line is, and how consistently it influences how you feel about yourself in everyday life. You also need to get an idea of how well your Action Plan helps you to deal with the times when your old Bottom Line resurfaces. It may be helpful to decide in advance when you will review how things are going and make any changes that seem helpful. Put reminders in your diary, or on your computer or smartphone.

Your Action Plan – The final draft

After a longer period of practice, review your Action Plan once again:

- How helpful has it been to you?
- How well did it keep you on track?
- Has it enabled you to continue to grow and develop?
- Has it helped you deal with setbacks in the best possible way?

If all is well, your second draft may be your final draft. If, on the other hand, your Action Plan still has shortcomings, you will need to make whatever changes are necessary, test-drive your new version for a limited period, and then review it again. When you are happy with it, make a clean copy, free of amendments, crossings-out and so on.

Remember that, unless you have superhuman powers to foretell the future, your Action Plan will never cover everything. However helpful it is, you should still be prepared to change and fine-tune it at any point in the future when you realise it could be extended or improved.

LOW SELF-ESTEEM: A Map of the Territory

(Early) Experience
Events, relationships, living conditions which have implications for your ideas
about yourself e.g. rejection; neglect; abuse; criticism and punishment;
lack of praise, interest, warmth; being the 'odd one out'

The Bottom Line
Assessment of your worth/value as a person
Conclusions about yourself, based on experience: *'This is the kind of person I am'*
e.g. *I am bad; I am worthless; I am stupid; I am not good enough*

Rules For Living
Guidelines, policies or strategies for getting by, given that you assume
the Bottom Line to be true
Standards against which self-worth can be measured e.g. *I must always put others first;*
If I say what I think, I will be rejected; Unless I do everything to the highest
possible standard, I will achieve nothing

Undermining the Negative Beliefs that Lie at the Heart of the Low Self-esteem:

(Early) Experience

The Bottom Line

Changing Unhelpful Rules For Living

Breaking the Vicious Circle

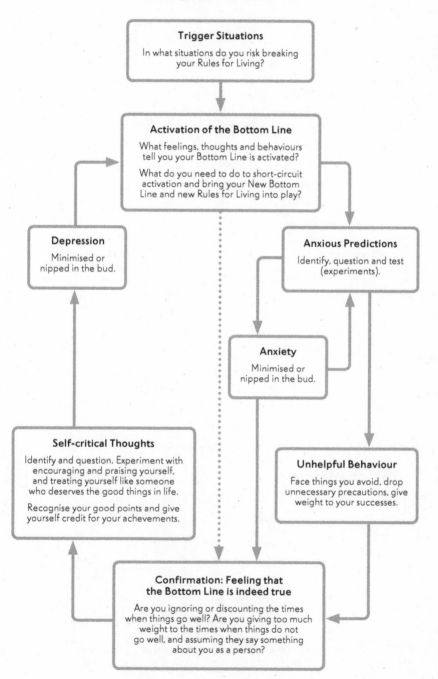

Breaking the Vicious Circle

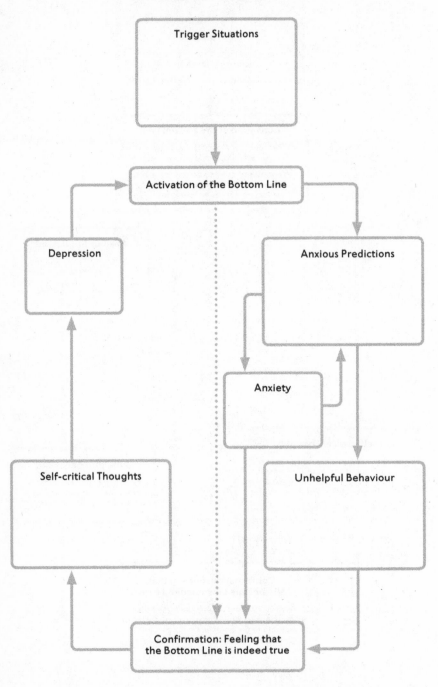

Fine-tuning your Action Plan: Getting SMART

Whichever stage you are at – first, second or final draft – make sure that your Action Plan meets the following **SMART** criteria. If your plan is not crystal clear, you may find after a few weeks that you are no longer certain what you are supposed to be doing. If your plan is too ambitious, you will not be able to carry it out successfully, and that could be demoralising. If on the other hand it is too limited, you may feel that you have stopped making progress. The **SMART** criteria will help you to ensure that your Action Plan takes you where you want to go.

ACTION PLANNING: SMART CRITERIA

Is it **SMART**?

Is it: **S**imple and **S**pecific enough?
Is it: **M**easurable?
Is it: **A**greed?
Is it: **R**ealistic?
Is the: **T**imescale reasonable?

S: Is it Simple and Specific enough?

Can you explain what you plan to do in words of one syllable? Is it so straightforward that even a child could understand it? To check this, try reading it out to a trusted friend or a member of your family. If they ask you to explain or clarify any of it, that part needs redrafting. When you have redrafted it, check out how it sounds to them.

M: Is it Measurable?

How will you know when you have achieved what you set out

to do? For example, in six months' time, if you have successfully acted on your Action Plan, how will you be feeling? Which of your new habits will still be in place? What specific targets will you have reached? How will you know that your New Bottom Line is still going strong? If you can specify clearly what you are going for, it will be much easier for you to judge how successfully you are putting your plan into practice, and to assess how helpful it is to you.

As you do this, beware of self-criticism sneaking in if your plan is not going as well as you wish or think it should. The point is to learn and develop your skills in consolidating and strengthening your new ways of operating, and of course this takes time and practice. You are learning new life skills and learning life skills is a lifelong process.

A: Is it Agreed?

Changes in you will mean changes for other people. For example, if you are planning to become more assertive about getting your needs met, then this will inevitably have an impact on those around you. If you are planning to change how you organise your working life (e.g. to reduce your working hours, in order to have more leisure time), then again this will have an impact on other people, both at work and at home.

When you make your Action Plan, it is important to take this into account. Do you need to communicate your intentions to others? Would it help to negotiate some of the changes you want with your family or friends? What about asking for help in sticking to your plan?

Even if you do not wish to involve others directly, consider what impact changes in you will have on them. Are they likely to react negatively in any way? What do you predict? You could, of course, be wrong – but you will be in a stronger position to stay on course if you have considered realistically what might happen and planned how you will deal with it (if necessary, with outside support).

Part of Briony's plan, for example, was to give herself more time to do things she enjoyed. She realised that she had allowed her family to get used to leaving all the housework to her. She decided that it would be a good idea to tell them about the work she had been doing to improve her self-esteem, and that she planned to start a fairer system of sharing the housework. She predicted that her family would see the justice of this, in theory, and would be in favour of what she was trying to do. She also predicted that, in practice, they would be reluctant to do their bit and would prefer to leave things as they were. So, in her plan, she included careful details of what to do when her family failed to change along with her. This included reminding herself of her reasons for making the change: she was a worthy person who deserved more out of life than to be a skivvy.

R: Is it Realistic?

When you plan ahead, take into account:

- Your state of emotional and physical health and fitness
- Your resources (e.g. money, time, people who care about and respect you)
- Other demands on your time and energy
- The level of support you have from friends, family, colleagues and others

Your Action Plan will be most solid and realistic if it takes these factors into account.

T: Is the Timescale reasonable?

Finally, make sure that you have considered carefully how much time you are willing to devote to putting your Action Plan into practice, and what timescale will allow you to achieve whatever targets you have set yourself. This may well include deciding what changes are most important to you, and which are less of a priority.

Ask yourself:

- What are your priorities? If you could complete only 20 per cent of your plan, which 20 per cent would you want it to be?
- If you believe it would still be helpful for you to record and question your thoughts regularly, how much time will you need to set aside every day for this?
- How much time might you need every week (or month) to assess how things are going and to set yourself new challenges?
- What are your personal objectives, as far as self-esteem is concerned (your milestones on the journey to healthy self-esteem)? Where do you want to be after three months? After six months? After one year?
- How frequently will you review your progress (successes, difficulties, what helped you, and what got in your way)?
- Have you set a date for your first review? This could be next week, or next month, or further away. Whenever it is, decide on a definite date and make an appointment with yourself. Make your review a special occasion. Take yourself out for lunch or give yourself a day out in the country, or at a health spa. At the very least, find a peaceful space in your home, and choose a time when you will not be interrupted, so that you can reflect on what you have achieved and think ahead.

Note the date and time for your review in your diary or on your calendar right now. And do not allow yourself to put it off. This is something you are doing for yourself. It is important. And you deserve it.

When drawing up your Action Plan ask yourself the Key Questions in the box on the next page.

KEY QUESTIONS

When Drawing up an Action Plan

1. How did my low self-esteem develop?
2. What kept it going?
3. What have I learned from this handbook?
4. What were my most important unhelpful thoughts, rules and beliefs? What alternatives did I find to them?
5. How can I build on what I have learned?
6. What might lead to a setback for me?
7. How will I know if all is not well? What are the early warning signs?
8. If I do have a setback, what will I do about it?

Let's take Briony's Action Plan for the Future as an example, using these key questions.

1 How did my low self-esteem develop?

When my parents died, I felt it was my fault. When my step-parents treated me so badly, that confirmed it. Finally, when my stepfather began to abuse me, I came to the conclusion that everything that had happened was a result of something in me. It all meant I was BAD. This was my Old Bottom Line. Once this idea was in place, other things happened that seemed to confirm it. For example, my first marriage was to a man who constantly criticised and ridiculed me. Because of what had happened earlier on, I thought this was just what I deserved.

2 What kept it going?

I kept on acting and thinking as if I really was a bad person. I never paid attention to good things about myself. I kept my true self hidden from people, because my Rule for Living was that if they found out what I was really like, they would want nothing further to do with me. I was always very hard on myself. Anything I got wrong filled me with despair – yet more evidence of what a bad person I was. I could not have close relationships, except with the few people who persisted even when I held back. I allowed people to dismiss me and treat me badly. I didn't think I deserved anything better.

3 What have I learned from this handbook?

To understand things better – it's my *belief* that I'm bad that's the problem, not that I really *am* bad. I have learned that it is possible to change beliefs about yourself that have been around for a long time, if you work on them. I have learned to still my critical voice and focus on the good things about me. I am changing my Rules and taking the risk of letting people see more of the true me.

4 What were my most important unhelpful thoughts, rules and beliefs? What alternatives did I find to them?

Unhelpful thought/rule/belief	*Alternative*
I am bad _____	I am worthy _____
If I let anyone get close to me, they will hurt and exploit me.	If I let people get close to me, I get the warmth and affection I need. Most people will treat me decently and I can protect myself from those who don't. Since my true self is worthy, I need not hide it. If some people don't like it, that's their problem.
I must never allow anyone to see my true self.	

5 How can I build on what I have learned? What do I need to do to ensure that my new ideas and skills become second nature, a routine part of how I go about my life?

Read the summary sheets for my new Rules and Bottom Line daily – I need to drum them in. Keep acting as if they were true and observe the results. When I notice myself getting anxious and wanting to avoid things or protect myself, work out what I am predicting and check it out. Watch out for self-criticism – it is deeply entrenched, and I need to keep fighting it. Keep on recording examples of good things about me – it has already made a difference. Make time for me – don't be afraid to remind the family when they go back to their old ways.

6 What might lead to a setback for me?

Getting depressed for any reason. Being consistently badly treated by someone. Something going very wrong for someone I cared about (I would tend to blame myself).

7 How will I know if all is not well? What are the early warning signs of a setback?

Wanting to shut myself away and avoid people. Getting snappy and irritable with my husband and children. Rise in tension, especially in my neck and shoulders.

8 If I do have a setback, what will I do about it?

Try to notice the early warning signals, for a start. Ask my husband to help with this – he's sensitive to when I start hiding myself away and being irritable and defensive, and he notices when I start being down on myself. Then get out my notes, especially the Summary Sheets and this Action Plan, and follow through on what I know works. Don't be hard on myself for taking a backward step – it's bound to happen from time to time, given how long I have felt bad about myself and how I came to be that way. Be encouraging and kind to myself, get all the support I can, and go back to the basics.

Now use the worksheet below to draw up your own **Action Plan for the Future.**

MY ACTION PLAN FOR THE FUTURE

1. **How did my low self-esteem develop?**

   Briefly summarise the experiences that led to the formation of your Old Bottom Line. Also include later experiences that have reinforced it, if they are relevant.

2. **What kept it going?**

   Briefly summarise your old unhelpful Rules for Living, and the thinking that fuelled your vicious circle (your anxious predictions and self-critical thoughts). What aspects of yourself did you home in on, or automatically screen out, ignore or discount? Finally, note the unnecessary precautions and self-defeating behaviour that prevented you from discovering that your predictions were not accurate and conspired to keep you down.

---

3. **What have I learned from this handbook?**

Make a note of the new ideas you have found most helpful (e.g. 'My beliefs about myself are opinions, not facts'). Also include particular methods you have learned for dealing with anxious and self-critical thoughts, Rules and beliefs about yourself (e.g. 'Review the evidence and look at the bigger picture', 'Don't assume, check it out'). Look back over what you have done and make a note of whatever you personally found most useful in practice.

4. **What were my most important unhelpful thoughts, Rules and beliefs about myself? What alternatives did I find to them?**

Write down the anxious predictions, self-critical thoughts, Rules for Living and Bottom Lines that caused you most trouble. Against each one, summarise the alternative you have discovered. You could use this format:

Unhelpful thought/ rule/belief	*Alternative*

5. **How can I build on what I have learned?**

Here is your opportunity to consider in detail what you need to do, in order to ensure that the new ideas and skills you have learned become second nature, a routine part of your life. It is also your chance to work out what changes you still want to make and use what you have learned to work on thoughts, Rules or beliefs about yourself you have not yet addressed. This may include going back to particular parts of this handbook and going through some sections again. It might also include further reading or deciding to seek help in order to take what you have discovered further or put it into practice more effectively (see pp. 409–414).

Ask yourself:

- Are there aspects of how your low self-esteem developed and what kept it going that you do not yet understand fully (Part One)? If so, how could you clarify them?

- Are there still situations where you feel anxious (Part Two, Section 1), but you are not clear why? Or situations where you understand very well what your anxious predictions are, but you have not yet faced them fully without dropping all your unnecessary precautions? If so, how will you use what you have learned to tackle these situations, and to deal with future anxieties?

- How will you ensure that you continue to spot and challenge self-critical thoughts (Part Two, Section 2)? What self-defeating behaviours do you still need to watch out for? What do you plan to do instead?

- How good are you at keeping your good points in mind and noticing examples of your qualities, strengths, skills and talents (Part Two, Section 3)? Do you still need to keep a written record? Even if you do not, might it be a useful resource to look over, if you have a setback at some point in the future?

- When you look at the pattern of your day and your week, are you achieving a good balance between 'A' activities (duties, obligations, tasks) and 'P' activities (pleasure, relaxation)?

If so, how will you ensure that you continue to do so? And if not, then how can you build on the changes you have already made?

- Are you routinely giving yourself credit for what you do and appreciating your achievements? If so, how can you ensure that you continue to do so? If not, why not – are self-critical thoughts creeping in, for example, or are you still hanging on to perfectionist standards? Whatever the reason, what do you need to do about it?

- How convincing do you now find your new Rules for Living (Part Three, Section 1)? What do you still need to do (if anything) to strengthen your belief in them and make acting on them second nature, even when the going gets tough? What experiments do you need to carry out? What thoughts are getting in your way, and how can you tackle them?

- How far are you now able to act as if your New Bottom Line was true? If you believe your New Bottom Line strongly and act routinely as if it was true, how can you ensure that it stays rock solid, even at times of pressure or distress?

6. **What might lead to a setback for me?**

   Consider what experiences or changes in your circumstances might still activate your Old Bottom Line and make you vulnerable to a setback. For example, supposing you were experiencing a high level of stress, or your life circumstances had become very difficult, or you were tired or unwell or upset for some other reason, this might still make you vulnerable to self-doubt. Working out what your own personal vulnerabilities might be will prepare you to notice quickly when things go wrong and do something about it.

7. **How will I know if all is not well? What are the early warning signs of a setback?**

   The first, essential thing is to notice what is happening. The early warning signs of a setback are unique to each person – like a fingerprint or signature. What clues would tell you that your Old Bottom Line was back in operation?

- How would you expect to feel?

- What might be going on in your body?

- What thoughts and images might run through your mind?

- What might you notice about your own behaviour (e.g. beginning to avoid challenges, dropping pleasurable activities, not standing up for yourself any more)?

- What might you notice in others (e.g. irritation, reassurance, apologies)?

The next thing is to consider in detail what to do if you spot the beginnings of a setback. How can you best care for yourself in this difficult situation, short-circuit the spiral down into low self-esteem, and make sure you get whatever support you need as you do so? How can you nip the setback in the bud?

Firstly, **DON'T PANIC!** It is quite natural to have setbacks on your journey towards overcoming low self-esteem, especially if the problem has been with you for a long time. Setbacks do not mean that you are back to square one, or that there is no point in doing anything further to help yourself. On the contrary, you simply need to return to what you have learned and begin putting it into practice regularly, until your self-esteem is back in balance. This may mean going back to basics (e.g. starting once again to record things regularly, perhaps after you have stopped needing to do so for some time). This is not a backward step. It is simply a sensible recognition that, for a limited period, you need to put in some extra time and effort to strengthen your New Bottom Line. Here are some questions to help you to think through how best to take care of yourself when you notice early warning signs.

8. **If I notice my Old Bottom Line coming back into operation, what will I do?**

- How will I respond when I notice early warning signs of a setback?

SUMMARY

1. The ideas and techniques you have learned from this handbook form a coherent programme for change.
2. To ensure that you carry forward what you have learned and make it part of your life, it is important to make a written Action Plan for the future.
3. Make your Action Plan straightforward and realistic. Ensure that you can measure your progress in carrying it out, and that it takes into account the impact of changes in you on those around you. It should also take account of limitations in your time and resources, and the time-scale should be realistic.
4. In your Action Plan, summarise your understanding of how your low self-esteem developed and what kept it going. Note what you have learned as you worked your way through the handbook, and how you plan to build on your new ideas and skills. Identify future events and stresses that might lead to a setback, and the early warning signs that would tell you all is not well. Then work out what to do and how best to take care of yourself if one occurs.

A Final Word of Encouragement

Congratulations on completing this Handbook. You have embarked on a journey of discovery and growth, investigating something central to your sense of who you are and the life you wish to lead. The work you have done can be challenging – the road may not be smooth or straightforward and often there are many ups and downs. Your persistence in this work is a statement of commitment to yourself, an acknowledgement of your worth, and an expression of compassion, courage and respect. You have explored what low self-esteem is, its impact, how it develops, and what keeps it going in the present day. You have learned how to weaken and dissolve old, self-defeating patterns of thinking and behaviour, and the unhelpful beliefs and rules that support them. And you have experimented with formulating and then living according to new, less negative, less rigid beliefs and rules which allow you to treat yourself just as you would treat a good friend, and to enjoy your life fully. Through this I hope that you have found new ways of relating to yourself with a greater sense of acceptance, ease, appreciation and kindness. I wish you well on your continuing journey towards lifelong healthy self-esteem.

THOUGHTS AND REFLECTIONS

THOUGHTS AND REFLECTIONS

Useful Books and Addresses

Useful Books

Ruth A. Baer, 2014. *Practising happiness: How mindfulness can free you from psychological traps and help you build the life you want.* Robinson.

David Burns, 2000. *Feeling Good: The new mood therapy.* Avon Books (2nd edition).

Gillian Butler, 2016. *Overcoming social anxiety and shyness: A self-help guide using cognitive-behavioural techniques.* Robinson (2nd edition).

Gillian Butler, Nick Grey and Tony Hope, 2018. *Manage Your Mind: The mental fitness guide.* Oxford University Press (2nd edition).

Paul Gilbert, 2009. *Overcoming Depression: A self-help guide using cognitive behavioural techniques.* Robinson (3rd edition).

Paul Gilbert, 2010. *The compassionate mind.* Robinson.

Dennis Greenberger and Christine A. Padesky, 2015. *Mind over mood: Change how you feel by changing the way you think.* Guilford Press (2nd edition).

Steven Hayes (with Spencer Smith), 2005. *Get out of your mind & into your life: The new acceptance and commitment therapy.* New Harbinger.

Helen Kennerley, 2009. *Overcoming childhood trauma: A self-help guide using cognitive behavioural techniques.* Robinson (2nd edition).

Helen Kennerley, 2014. *Overcoming anxiety: A self-help guide using cognitive behavioural techniques*. Robinson (2nd edition).

Matthew McKay and Patrick Fanning, 2016. *Self-esteem: A proven program of cognitive techniques for assessing, improving, and maintaining your self-esteem*. New Harbinger (4th edition).

Roz Shafran, Sarah Egan and Tracey Wade, 2018. *Overcoming perfectionism: A self-help guide using cognitive behavioural techniques*. Robinson (2nd edition).

Mary Welford, 2012. *Building your self-confidence using compassion focused therapy*. Robinson.

Mark Williams and Danny Penman, 2011. *Mindfulness: A practical guide to finding peace in a frantic world*. Piatkus.

Website: Reading Well for Mental Health (makes mental health self-help books freely available via local libraries) https://reading-well.org.uk

Useful addresses

GREAT BRITAIN

British Association for Behavioural Cognitive Psychotherapies
Imperial House
Hornby Street,
Bury, Lancashire BL9 5BM

Tel: (0044) 161 705 4304
Website: www.babcp.com

British Association for Counselling & Psychotherapy
BACP House
15 St John's Business Park
Lutterworth, Leicestershire LE17 4HB

Tel: (0044) 1455 883300
Website: www.bacp.co.uk

British Psychological Society
St Andrews House
48 Princess Road East
Leicester LE1 7DR

Tel: (0044) 116 254 9568
Website: www.bps.org.uk

Mental Health Foundation (Headquarters)
Colechurch House
1 London Bridge Walk
London SE1 2SX

Tel: (0044) 20 7803 1100
Website: www.mentalhealth.org.uk

MIND: The National Association for Mental Health
15–19 Broadway
Stratford
London E15 4BQ

Tel: (0044) 20 8519 2122
Website: www.mind.org.uk

Newcastle Cognitive & Behavioural Therapies Centre
Benfield House
Walkergate Park
Benfield Road
Newcastle upon Tyne, NE6 4PF

Tel: (0044) 191 287 6100
Website: www.ntw.nhs.uk

Oxford Cognitive Therapy Centre
Warneford Hospital
Oxford OX3 7JX

Tel: (0044) 1865 902801
Website: www.octc.co.uk

AUSTRALIA

Australian Association for Cognitive & Behaviour Therapy
AACBT Ltd
15 Haig Avenue
Georges Hall
New South Wales NSW 2198

Website: www.aabct.org.au

Australian Centre for Clinical Interventions
223 James Street
Northbridge
Western Australia 6003

Tel: (0061) 08 9227 4399
Website: www.cci.health.wa.gov.au

CANADA

Canadian Association of Cognitive & Behavioural Therapies
CACBT-ACTCC
260 Queen Street West
PO Box 60055
Toronto, ON
M5V 0C5

Website: www.cacbt.ca

EUROPE

European Association of Behavioural & Cognitive Therapies
EABCT Office
PO Box 14081
3508 SC Utrecht, The Netherlands

Tel: (0031) 30 254 30 54
Website: www.eabct.eu

NEW ZEALAND

Aotearoa New Zealand Association for Cognitive Behavioural Therapies

Website: www.cbt.org.nz

UNITED STATES

Academy of Cognitive Therapy
245 N. 15th Street, MS 403
17 New College Building
Department of Psychiatry
Philadelphia, PA 19102

Tel: (001) 215 831 7838
Website: www.academyofct.org

American Institute for Cognitive Therapy
136 E. 57th Street, Suite 1101
New York City, NY 10022

Tel: (001) 212 308 2440
Website: www.cognitivetherapynyc.com

The Association for Behavioral & Cognitive Therapies (ABCT)
305 7th Avenue, 16th Floor
New York, NY 10001

Tel: (001) 212 647 1890
Website: www.abct.org

Institute for Behavior Therapy
20 E. 49th Street, 2nd Floor
New York, NY 10017

Tel: (001) 212 692 9288
Website: www.ifbt.com

Extra Charts and Worksheets

(Found in Part One, Section 1)

HOW DOES LOW SELF-ESTEEM AFFECT A PERSON?

Think of a recent meeting with someone you know who you consider to have low self-esteem:

1. **What did you talk about?** (For example, did you hear lots of apologies, or a lot of self-criticism, self-blame or self-doubt?)

_____

_____

_____

_____

2. **How did the person behave?** (Did he or she sit hunched over, looking down? Did he or she speak in a hushed voice, or avoid making eye contact? Or did you perhaps have the feeling he or she was putting on a front – working hard to appear cheerful, for example, or trying too hard to please instead of relaxing and being natural?)

_____

_____

_____

_____

---

3. **What sort of mood was the person in?** (For example, did he or she seem sad, shy, anxious, ashamed, hopeless, frustrated or angry?)

_____

_____

_____

_____

4. **How was the person's body state?** (For example, did he or she seem tired, low in energy, restless or tense?)

_____

_____

_____

_____

(Found in Part One, Section 2)

Biased perception (focusing on weaknesses and ignoring strengths)

Think back over the last week or two and write down three occasions when you focused on a weakness or ignored a strength:

1. _____

_____

_____

_____

_____

_____

2. _____

_____

_____

_____

_____

3. _____

_____

_____

_____

_____

Biased interpretation (always seeing the downside)

Write down three recent occasions when you twisted something that happened to fit your negative view of yourself:

1. _____
   _____
   _____
   _____
   _____
   _____

2. _____
   _____
   _____
   _____
   _____

3. _____
   _____
   _____
   _____
   _____

(Found in Part One, Section 2)

RULES FOR LIVING

- What are your Rules for Living?

_____

_____

_____

_____

_____

_____

- Think about your Rules and write down how each one helps you in life.

_____

_____

_____

_____

_____

_____

_____

_____

- Now write down how each Rule restricts you in your
  life.

_____

_____

_____

_____

_____

_____

_____

_____

Anxious vicious circle

Trigger Situation

Situation where you fear your Rule *might* be broken

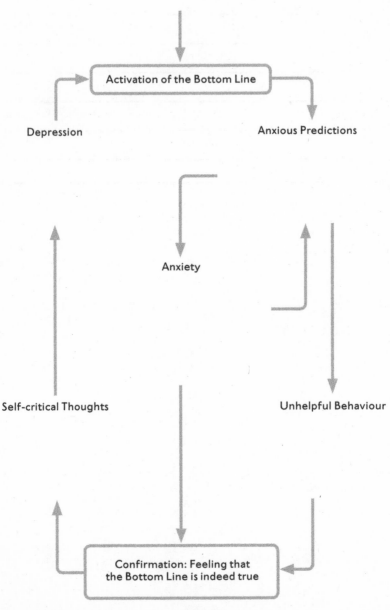

Activation of the Bottom Line

Depression

Anxious Predictions

Anxiety

Self-critical Thoughts

Unhelpful Behaviour

Confirmation: Feeling that
the Bottom Line is indeed true

Anxious vicious circle

Trigger Situation

Situation where you fear your Rule *might* be broken

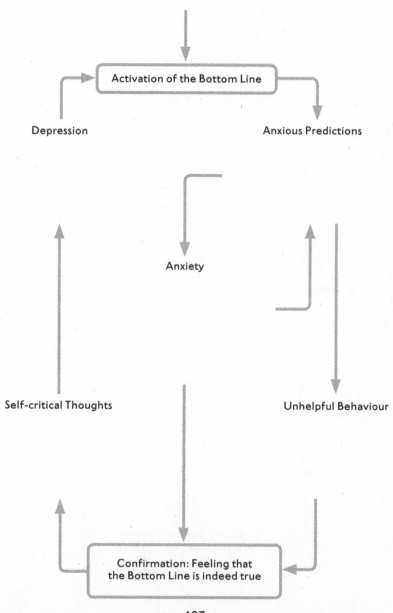

Activation of the Bottom Line

Depression

Anxious Predictions

Anxiety

Self-critical Thoughts

Unhelpful Behaviour

Confirmation: Feeling that
the Bottom Line is indeed true

Depressed vicious circle

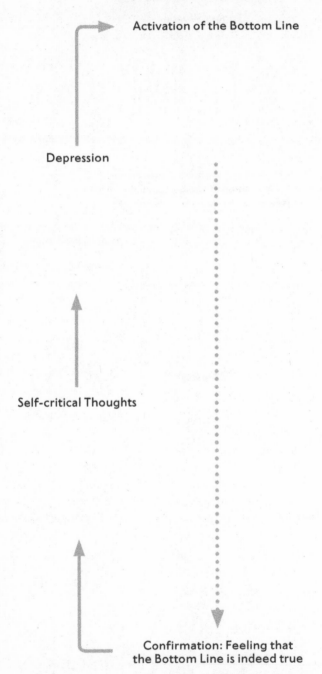

Activation of the Bottom Line

Depression

Self-critical Thoughts

Confirmation: Feeling that
the Bottom Line is indeed true

Depressed vicious circle

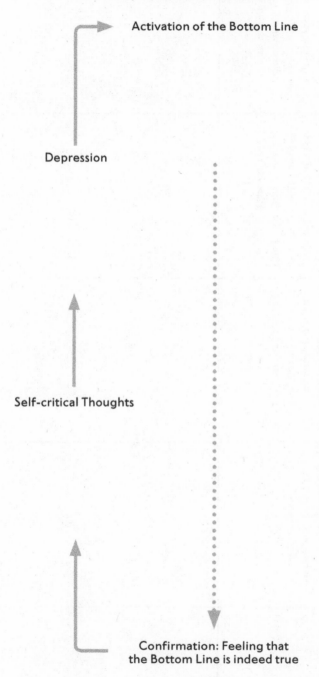

Activation of the Bottom Line

Depression

Self-critical Thoughts

Confirmation: Feeling that
the Bottom Line is indeed true

Predictions and Precautions Chart

Date/Time	Situation What were you doing when you began to feel anxious?	Emotions and body sensations (e.g. anxious, panicky, tense, heart racing). Rate 0–100 for intensity.	Anxious predictions What exactly was going through your mind when you began to feel anxious (e.g. thoughts in words, images)? Rate each one 0–100% for how far you believed it.	Precautions What did you do to stop your predictions coming true (e.g. avoid the situation, take precautions)?

Questioning Anxious Predictions Chart

Date/Time	Situation	Emotions and body sensations Rate 0–100% for intensity.	Anxious predictions Rate belief 0–100%.	Alternative perspectives Use the key questions to find other views of the situation. Rate belief 0–100%.	Outcome 1. What did you do instead of taking your usual precautions? 2. What were the results? 3. What did you learn?

Using Experiments to Check Out Anxious Predictions Chart

Date/Time	Situation	Anxious predictions Rate belief 0–100%.	Experiment What will I do instead of taking precautions?	Results 1. What have you learned? 2. Were your predictions correct? If not, what perspective would make better sense?

Spotting Self-Critical Thoughts Chart

Date/Time	Situation	Emotions and body sensations	Self-critical thoughts	Unhelpful behaviour
	What were you doing when you began to feel bad about yourself?	(e.g. sad, angry, guilty, tense). Rate each 0–100 for intensity.	What exactly was going through your mind when you began to feel bad about yourself (e.g. thoughts in words, images, meanings)? Rate belief in each one 0–100%.	What did you do as a consequence of your self-critical thoughts?

Questioning Self-Critical Thoughts Chart

Date/Time	Situation	Emotions and body sensations Rate each 0–100 for intensity.	Self-critical thoughts Rate belief in each 0–100%.	Alternative perspectives Use the key questions to find other perspectives on yourself. Rate belief in each one 0–100%..	Outcome 1. Now that you have found alternatives to your self-critical thoughts, how do you feel (0–100)? 2. How far do you now believe the self-critical thoughts (0–100%)? 3. What can you do (action plan, experiments)?

Good Points Chart		
Date/Time	What I did	Positive quality

Good Points Chart		
Date/Time	What I did	Positive quality

Daily Activity Diary		Monday	Tuesday	Wednesday	Thursday	Friday	Saturday	Sunday
M O R N I N G	6–7							
	7–8							
	8–9							
	9–10							
	10–11							
	11–12							

12–1	1–2	2–3	3–4	4–5

AFTERNOON

	Monday	Tuesday	Wednesday	Thursday	Friday	Saturday	Sunday
5–6							
6–7							
7–8							
8–9							
9–10							
10–11							

EVENING

11–12	
12–1	

Review: (What do you notice about your day? What worked for you? What did not work? What would you like to change?)

Mon:

Tues:

Weds:

Thurs:

Fri:

Sat:

Sun:

Daily Activity Diary		Monday	Tuesday	Wednesday	Thursday	Friday	Saturday	Sunday
M O R N I N G	6–7							
	7–8							
	8–9							
	9–10							
	10–11							
	11–12							

12–1	1–2	2–3	3–4	4–5
AFTERNOON				

	Monday	Tuesday	Wednesday	Thursday	Friday	Saturday	Sunday
5–6							
6–7							
7–8							
8–9							
9–10							
10–11							

EVENING

	11–12	12–1

Review: (What do you notice about your day? What worked for you? What did not work? What would you like to change?)

Mon:

Tues:

Weds:

Thurs:

Fri:

Sat:

Sun:

RULES FOR LIVING DOWNWARD ARROW CHART

Situation:_____

Emotions: _____

Key thought:_____

What does this mean to you?

↓

_____

_____

↓

And if that was true, what would it mean to you?

↓

_____

_____

↓

And supposing that happened, what would it mean to you?

↓

_____

_____

↓

And what would that mean to you?

↓

_____

_____

↓

So, what's the Rule?

↓

_____

_____

CHANGING THE RULES: MY SUMMARY

1. My old Rule is:

2. This Rule has had the following impact on my life:

3. I know that the Rule is in operation because:

4. It is understandable that I have this Rule, because:

5. However, the Rule is unreasonable, because:

6. The advantages of obeying the Rule are:

7. But the disadvantages are:

8. A more realistic and helpful Rule would be:

9. In order to test-drive the new Rule, I need to:

Experimenting with New Rules Worksheet

Date/time	The situation	What I did	The outcome (what I noticed, felt, thought, learned)

BOTTOM LINE DOWNWARD ARROW CHART

Situation:_____

Emotions: _____

Key thought:_____

What does that mean about me?

↓

_____

_____

↓

What does that mean about me?

↓

_____

_____

↓

What does that mean about me?

↓

_____

_____

↓

What does that mean about me?

↓

_____

_____

↓

So I am:

↓

_____

_____

Acting in Accordance with my New Bottom Line

Date/Time	Experiment (what I did)	Results (what I noticed, my feelings, sensations and thoughts, others' reactions, what I learned)	My belief in my Old Bottom Line	My belief in my New Bottom Line

BOTTOM LINE WORKSHEET

When you have rated your degree of belief, take a moment to focus on your Bottom Line and notice what feelings emerge. Write down any emotions you experience (e.g. sadness, anger, guilt), and rate them according to how powerful they are (from 0 to 100). Again, you may notice that, although you can still call up your Bottom Line, your feelings when you focus on it are less intense.

My Old Bottom Line is: 'I am _____

_____ ,

                                      Belief   Emotions (0–100)

When the Old Bottom
  Line is most convincing: _____ %.

When it is least convincing: _____ %.

When I started the book: _____ %.

My New Bottom Line is: 'I am _____

_____ ,

                                        Belief   Emotions (0–100)

When the New Bottom
  Line is most convincing: _____ %.

When it is least convincing: _____ %.

When I started the book: _____ %.

'Evidence' supporting the Old Bottom Line and how I now understand it:

'Evidence'   **New Understanding**

In the light of my new understanding,
  I now believe my Old Bottom Line: _____ %
In the light of my new understanding,
  I now believe my New Bottom Line: _____ %

Evidence (past and present) which supports my New Bottom Line:

_____

_____

_____

_____

_____

In the light of this evidence,
   I now believe my Old Bottom Line: _____ %
In the light of this evidence,
   I now believe my New Bottom Line: _____ %

Observation: Information and experiences I need to be alert to, in order to gather more evidence to support my New Bottom Line:

_____

_____

_____

_____

_____

_____

Experiments: Specific things I need to do, in order to gather more evidence to support my New Bottom Line:

_____

_____

_____

_____

_____

Undermining the Negative Beliefs that Lie at the Heart of the Low Self-esteem:

(Early) Experience

The Bottom Line

Changing Unhelpful Rules For Living

Breaking the Vicious Circle

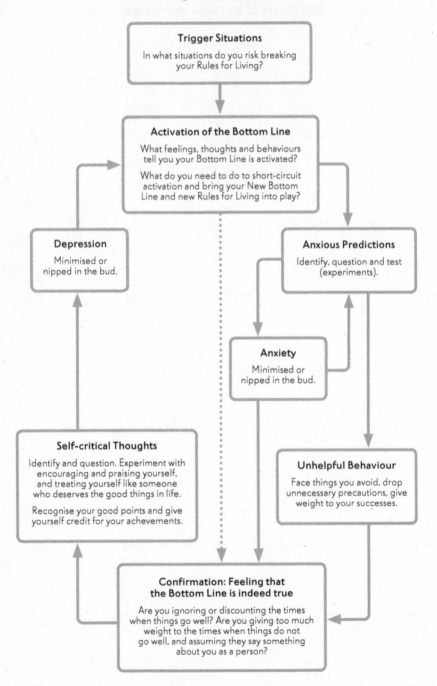

Trigger Situations

In what situations do you risk breaking your Rules for Living?

Activation of the Bottom Line

What feelings, thoughts and behaviours tell you your Bottom Line is activated?

What do you need to do to short-circuit activation and bring your New Bottom Line and new Rules for Living into play?

Depression

Minimised or nipped in the bud.

Anxious Predictions

Identify, question and test (experiments).

Anxiety

Minimised or nipped in the bud.

Self-critical Thoughts

Identify and question. Experiment with encouraging and praising yourself, and treating yourself like someone who deserves the good things in life.

Recognise your good points and give yourself credit for your achevements.

Unhelpful Behaviour

Face things you avoid, drop unnecessary precautions, give weight to your successes.

Confirmation: Feeling that the Bottom Line is indeed true

Are you ignoring or discounting the times when things go well? Are you giving too much weight to the times when things do not go well, and assuming they say something about you as a person?

THOUGHTS AND REFLECTIONS

THOUGHTS AND REFLECTIONS

Thanks

Heartfelt thanks to all the colleagues (and friends) who have expanded my thinking and opened my mind to new discoveries, and from whom I have learned so much. Especially Aaron T. Beck, John Teasdale, Gillian Butler, David Clark, Anke Ehlers, Paul Salkovskis, Christine Padesky, Kathleen Mooney, Ann Hackmann, Joan Kirk, Mark Williams, John Peacock, Ferris Urbanowski and Jon Kabat-Zinn. My thanks, too, to all the patients with whom I have been privileged to spend time over the years. And to the staff at Robinson (and especially Andrew McAleer) for their encouragement and their expertise. And above all, to my family – Clive, Emily and Jacob.

Index

457

an **OVERCOMING** publication

an introduction to

Improving your Self-Esteem

Second Edition

Melanie **Fennell**
Lee **Brosan**

An Introduction to Improving Your Self-Esteem

2nd Edition

Practical support for overcoming low self-esteem

Low self-esteem can impact on many areas of your life such as your relationships, work life and general wellbeing. This invaluable self-help guide will help you to understand what has led to your poor self-esteem, what keeps it going and how to improve your self-image, gaining a more balanced and positive view of yourself.

This book is based on clinically proven cognitive behavioural therapy (CBT) techniques to help you improve your confidence. You will learn:

- How low self-esteem develops
- How to challenge negative predictions
- How to improve self-acceptance

OVERCOMING

Low
Self-Esteem

2nd Edition

A self-help guide
using cognitive
behavioural techniques

MELANIE FENNELL

an
OVERCOMING
publication

READING
WELL

Overcoming Low Self-Esteem

2nd Edition

A self-help guide using cognitive behavioural techniques

Boost your confidence and change your life for the better

Low self-esteem can make life difficult in all sorts of ways. It can make you anxious and unhappy, tormented by doubts and self-critical thoughts. It can get in the way of feeling at ease with other people and stop you from leading the life you want to lead. It makes it hard to value and appreciate yourself in the same way you would another person you care about.

Melanie Fennell's acclaimed and bestselling self-help guide will help you to understand your low self-esteem and break out of the vicious circle of distress, unhelpful behaviour and self-destructive thinking. Using practical techniques from Cognitive Behavioural Therapy (CBT), this book will help you learn the art of self-acceptance and so transform your sense of yourself for the better.

Specifically, you will learn:

- How low self-esteem develops and what keeps it going
- How to question your negative thoughts and the attitudes that underlie them
- How to identify your strengths and good qualities for a more balanced, kindly view of yourself

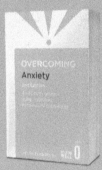
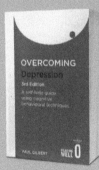
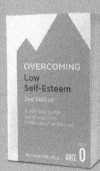